D0662930

On Behalf of ICDRG

Springer
Berlin
Heidelberg
New York
Hong Kong
London
Milan
Paris
Tokyo

J.-M. Lachapelle · H. I. Maibach

Patch Testing and Prick Testing

A Practical Guide

With a Contribution by J. Ring

With 37 Color Figures
and 42 Tables

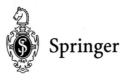

Springer

Professor Jean-Marie Lachapelle
Department of Dermatology
Louvain University
UCL 3033
30 Clos Chapelle-aux-Champs
1200 Brussels, Belgium

Professor Johannes Ring
Klinik und Poliklinik
für Dermatologie und Allergologie
am Biederstein der Technischen
Universität München
Biedersteinerstr. 29
80802 München, Germany

Professor Howard I. Maibach
Department of Dermatology
University of California
San Francisco School of Medicine
Box 0989
Surge 110
San Francisco, CA 94143-0989, USA

ISBN 3-540-44349-5 Springer-Verlag Berlin Heidelberg New York

Cataloging-in-Publication Data applied for

A catalog record for this book is available from the Library of Congress.

Bibliographic information published by Die Deutsche Bibliothek
Die Deutsche Bibliothek lists this publication in the Deutsche Nationalbibliografie;
detailed bibliographic data is available in the Internet at http://dnb.ddb.de

Springer-Verlag Berlin Heidelberg New York
a member of BertelsmannSpringer Science+Business Media GmbH

http://www.springer.de

© Springer-Verlag Berlin Heidelberg 2003
Printed in Germany

Cover design: Erich Kirchner, Heidelberg
Typesetting: Fotosatz-Service Köhler GmbH, Würzburg
Printing and bookbinding: Stürtz AG, Würzburg
Printed on acid-free paper   24/3150PF   5 4 3 2 1 0

Preface

This small book is a follow-up to the classic *Manual of Contact Dermatitis* by Siegfried Fregert, which was published on behalf of the International Contact Dermatitis Research Group and the North American Contact Dermatitis Group.

The format follows the succinct presentation of Professor Fregert. Every emphasis has been made on balancing brevity and clarity with sufficient details for the beginner in the field of diagnostic patch and prick testing.

Brevity is valued by the beginner. Fortunately, several major textbooks including those by Cronin, Kanerva, Rycroft, and Fisher are available and provide for the second level of detail.

The authors would greatly appreciate any corrections and suggestions – for future editions.

J.-M. Lachapelle
H.-I. Maibach

Contents

Abbreviations

ACD	Allergic contact dermatitis
ACDS	Allergic contact dermatitis syndrome
AD	Atopic dermatitis
AE	Atopic eczema
APT	Atopy patch test
BCEDG	Belgian Contact and Environmental Dermatitis Group
CAD	Chronic actinic dermatitis
CADR	Cutaneous adverse drug reactions
CR	Current relevance
CUS	Contact urticaria syndrome
EECDRG	European and Environmental Contact Dermatitis Research Group
ESCD	European Society of Contact Dermatitis
ESS	Excited skin syndrome (angry back)
ETFAD	European Task Force on Atopic Dermatitis
FDA	Food and Drug Administration
ICDRG	International Contact Dermatitis Research Group
ICU	Immunological contact urticaria
IFRA	International Fragrance Association
IgE	Immunoglobulin E
JCDS	Japanese Society for Contact Dermatitis
MED	Minimum erythema dose
NACDG	North American Contact Dermatitis Research Group
NICU	Non-immunological contact urticaria
PACD	Photoallergic contact dermatitis
PCD	Protein contact dermatitis
PLE	Polymorphic light eruption
PNU	Protein nitrogen units

PR	Past relevance
PUT	Provocative use test
RAST	Radioallergosorbent test
ROAT	Repeated open application test
SRCD	Systemic reactivation of contact dermatitis
UVL	Ultraviolet light

CHAPTER 1

The International Contact Dermatitis Research Group

J.-M. LACHAPELLE, H. I. MAIBACH

1.1
Historical Background

The International Contact Dermatitis Research Group (ICDRG) was founded in 1967. It was (and still is) an informal association, without any statutes.

The founding members of the group were 11: C.D. Calnan, E. Cronin, D.S. Wilkinson (United Kingdom); N. Hjorth (Denmark); V. Pirilä (Finland), H.J. Bandmann (Germany); C.L. Meneghini (Italy); K.E. Malten (Holland); S. Fregert, and B. Magnusson (Sweden). Niels Hjorth acted as Chairman of the Group.

The main aim of the group was to provide a standardization of Routine Patch Testing [1]. This standardization did not exist at the time. "As long as clinics used different techniques, substances, concentrations and vehicles for testing, results obtained at various clinics in different countries could not be compared" [2]. The members of the ICDRG conducted several extensive joint studies, and this resulted in the production of the so-called ICDRG standard series, known and used throughout the world.

The ICDRG promoted the foundation of several contact dermatitis national and international groups. This goal was reached in the 1980s [3].

Some groups, e.g. the European and Environmental Contact Dermatitis Research Group (EECDRG) and the North American Contact Dermatitis Group (NACDG) took over the task of standardization of various series of allergens. A similar task was achieved in different countries by national groups, which tried to adapt series of tests to local needs, in relationship with the specific environment encountered in each individual country.

1.2
Current Tasks of the ICDRG

The current tasks adopted by the present ICDRG committee are the following:

- To promote the dissemination of our knowledge in the field of environmental dermatology (with a special interest in contact dermatitis). This goal is reached by the organization of international symposia (on a 2-year schedule). The aim of the symposia is to allow dermatologists, occupational physicians, chemists and pharmacists to be acquainted with up-dated information. The symposia are organized in different parts of the world.
- To promote the publication of manuals which are of practical use for practising dermatologists and occupational physicians.

1.3
ICDRG Members

Chairman   Prof. J.-M. Lachapelle, Department of Dermatology, Louvain University, UCL 3033, 30 Clos Chapelle-aux-Champs, 1200 Brussels, Belgium; Tel.: +32-2-7643335, Fax: +32-2-7643334, e-mail: Jean-marie.Lachapelle@derm.ucl.ac.be

Secretary   Prof. R. Hayakawa, Department of Environmental Dermatology, Nagoya University School of Medicine, 1–1-20 Daikominami, Higashi-ku, Nagoya 4610047, Japan; Tel.: +81-52-7191983, Fax: +81-52-7191984, e-mail: hayakawa@med.nagoya-u.ac.jp

Members   Prof. I. Ale, Department of Dermatology, Hospital de Clinicas "Dr. Manuel Quintela", 11300 Montevideo, Uruguay; Tel.: +598-2-472571, Fax: +598-2-473182, e-mail: irisale@apolo.hc.edu.uy

Prof. P.U. Elsner, Department of Dermatology, Friedrich-Schiller University, Erfurter Strasse 35, 07740 Jena, Germany; Tel.: +49-3641-937370, Fax : +49-3641-937418, e-mail: elsner@derma.uni-jena.de

Prof. H.C. Eun, Department of Dermatology, Seoul National University College of Medicine, 28, Chongo-gu, Yungon-dong, Seoul 110–744, Korea; Tel.: +82-2-7602415, Fax: +82-2-7455934, e-mail: hceun@snu.ac.be

Dr. S. Freeman, Skin and Cancer Foundation, Contact and Occupational Clinic, 277 Bourke Street, Darlinghurst, NSW 2010, Australia; Tel.: +61-2-93604480, Fax: +61-2-93311244, e-mail: suron@enternet.com.au

Prof. C.L. Goh, National Skin Centre, 1 Mandalay Road, 1130 Singapore, Singapore; Tel.: +65-3508471, Fax: +65-2533225, e-mail: nsc@pacific.net.sg

Prof. M. Hannuksela, South Karelia Central Hospital, Käkelänkatu 4A, 53130 Lappeenranta, Finland; Tel.: +358-53-5315610, Fax: +358-5-6115699, e-mail: matti.hannuksela@ekshp.fi

Prof. L. Kanerva, Section of Dermatology, Finnish Institute of Occupational Health, Topeliuksenkatu 41A, 00250 Helsinki, Finland; Tel.: +358-9-4747288, Fax: +358-9-2413691

Prof. H.I. Maibach, Department of Dermatology, University of California, San Francisco School of Medicine, Box 0989, Surge 110, San Francisco, CA 94143–0989, USA; Tel.: +1-415-4762468, Fax: +1-415-7535304, e-mail: himjlm@itsa.UCSF.edu

Prof. J. Wahlberg, Department of Occupational and Environmental Dermatology, Karolinska Hospital, 17176 Stockholm, Sweden; Tel.: +46-8-51773629, Fax: +46-8-344445, e-mail: jan.Wahlberg@smd.sll.se

References

1. Lachapelle JM (2001) Historical aspects. In: Rycroft RJG, Menné T, Frosch PJ, Lepoittevin JP (eds) Textbook of contact dermatitis, 3rd edn. Springer, Berlin, pp 1–10
2. Calnan CD, Fregert S, Magnusson B (1976) The International Contact Dermatitis Research Group. Cutis 18:708–710
3. Bruynzeel DP (2001) Contact Dermatitis Research Groups. In: Rycroft RJG, Menné T, Frosch PJ, Lepoittevin JP (eds) Textbook of contact dermatitis, 3rd edn. Springer, Berlin, pp 1029–1035

**Part 1
Patch Testing**

CHAPTER 2

The Spectrum of Diseases for Which Patch Testing Is Recommended

Patients Who Should Be Investigated

J.-M. LACHAPELLE

Textbooks of dermatology claim that patch testing is the "tool" of investigation for patients presenting (or having presented) with symptoms of allergic contact dermatitis (ACD). The aim of the procedure is to "trap" one or several suspected contact allergen(s) (see Sect. 3.2). This classical view is restrictive in many respects, and requires broadening in order to fulfil its real diagnostic interest. Therefore, the use of patch testing is expanded to a wide spectrum of skin conditions. We recommend it in the following situations; (a) in all clinical stages of the allergic contact dermatitis syndrome (ACDS) as explained in Sect. 2.2; and (b) in various skin diseases (mainly but not exclusively eczematous) in which ACD may be superimposed, as detailed in Sect. 2.3. A special section is devoted to hand dermatitis (see Sect. 2.4), the importance of which is considered notorious in daily practice.

2.1
Allergic Contact Dermatitis

Allergic contact dermatitis (ACD) is a classic delayed-type hypersensitivity, or a type IV immunological reaction, that occurs in two phases, initially a sensitization and then an elicitation response.

2.1.1
Sensitization Phase

The allergen is a chemical that is usually, but not always, of low molecular weight, lipid-soluble, and highly reactive. An unprocessed allergen is more correctly referred to as a hapten. The hapten is applied to the stratum corneum, penetrates to the lower layers of the epidermis, and is taken up by the Langerhans' cell by pinocytosis. Within the cell, lyosomal or cytosolic enzymes chemically alter the hapten, and it is conjugated to a newly synthesized HLA-DR molecule to form the complete antigen. This complex is expressed on the surface of the Langerhans' cell.

The Langerhans' cell exists in a resting or immature state and in that state functions primarily as a macrophage with little ability to stimulate T cells. When the skin is exposed to allergens, the keratinocytes secrete cytokines that produce maturation of the Langerhans' cell to an activated state, which allows them to stimulate T cells. This activation alters the phenotype of the Langerhans' cell with upregulation of secretion of certain cytokines and expression of various cell surface molecules, including class I and II MHC, ICAM-1, LFA-3, and B7.

The next step in the process is the presentation of the HLA-DR-antigen complex to specific helper T cells that express both a CD4 molecule that recognizes the HLA-DR of the Langerhans' cells and more specifically a T-cell receptor CD3 complex that recognizes the processed antigen. There is some evidence that antigen can also be presented in the context of the MHC class I molecules, in which case it would be recognized by CD8 cells.

It is believed that the Langerhans' cell migrates via the lymphatics to regional nodes, where it presents the HLA-DR-antigen complex to specific T cells. Once antigen recognition occurs, both cells are activated. A series of cytokines is synthesized by both the Langerhans' cell and the T cell. Within the T cell, this message is transmitted via the CD3 molecule. The Langerhans' cell secretes interleukin (IL)-1, which stimulates the T cell to secrete IL-2 and to express IL-2 receptors. This cytokine leads to stimulation of T-cell proliferation, thereby expanding the clone of specific T cells capable of responding to the inciting antigen. This occurs during the classic lag phase of sensitization. The primed or memory T cells that are generated are now much expanded compared with the original population of cells with the specific T-cell receptor, and they leave the node and circulate throughout the body. The individual is now sensitized, or primed, to respond when these circulating T cells are re-exposed to antigen.

2.1.2
Elicitation Phase

The second phase, or elicitation of the delayed type of hypersensitivity, occurs on re-exposure. Once again, hapten diffuses to the Langerhans' cell, it is taken in and chemically altered, it is bound to the HLA-DR, and the complex is expressed on the surface of the Langerhans' cell. The complex interacts with primed T cells in the skin or the node (or both), and the activation process takes place. In the skin the interaction is even more complex because other cells are present; Langerhans' cells secrete IL-1, which stimulates the T cell to produce IL-2 and express IL-2R. Once again, this leads to proliferation and expansion of the T-cell population, this time within the skin. In addition, the activated T cells secrete IFN-γ, which activates the keratinocyte and causes it to express both ICAM-1 and HLA-DR. The ICAM-1 molecule allows the keratinocyte to interact with T cells and other leucocytes that express the LFA-1 molecule. Expression of HLA-DR allows for the keratinocyte to interact directly with CD-4-bearing T cells and may allow for antigen presentation to these cells as well. In addition, HLA-DR expression may make the keratinocyte the target for cytotoxic T cells. Activated keratinocytes also produce a number of cytokines, including IL-1, IL-6, and GMCSF, all of which can further expand the involvement and activation of T cells. In addition, IL-1 can stimulate keratinocytes to produce eicosanoids. This combination of cytokines and eicosanoids leads to activation of mast cells and macrophages. Histamine from mast cells and eicosanoids from mast cells, keratinocytes, and infiltrating leucocytes lead to vascular dilation and increased permeability to circulating proinflammatory soluble factors and cells. This cascade leads to the clinical ACD response of inflammation, cellular destruction, and reparative processes.

2.1.3
Clinical Symptoms

ACD can produce an acute eczematous picture with vesicles and weeping (Fig. 2.1); subacute eczema with erythema, scaling, juicy papules, and weeping; and chronic eczema with hyperkeratosis, fissuring, and lichenification.

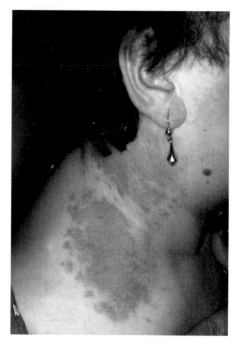

Fig. 2.1. Allergic contact dermatitis to paraphenylenediamine from a permanent hair dye

This distinction among acute, subacute, and chronic may be chronological and evolve from one to another.

We emphasize that clinical symptoms of ACD are usually straightforward; nevertheless, in some instances (see Sect. 2.2.1, Morphological Aspects) clinical diagnosis may be less evident, since distinctive features between irritant and allergic contact dermatitis are not always obvious. In these cases, patch testing is an undisputed tool for clarifying the situation. ACD is stage 1 (see Sect. 2.2.1) of the allergic contact dermatitis syndrome, described in full detail in the following section.

2.2
The Allergic Contact Dermatitis Syndrome

We recently developed the concept of the allergic contact dermatitis syndrome (ACDS) [1]. A syndrome can be defined as a group of signs and symptoms that actively indicate or characterize a disease [2].

A similar approach was made previously in the literature regarding irritation, i.e. the irritant contact dermatitis syndrome [3], and contact urticaria, i.e. the contact urticaria syndrome [4]. The concept of ACDS considers the various facets of contact allergy, including morphological aspects and staging by symptomatology.

The three stages of ACDS can be defined as follows:

Stage 1. The skin symptoms are limited to the site(s) of application of contact allergen(s).

Stage 2. There is a regional dissemination of symptoms (via lymphatic vessels), extending from the site of application of allergen(s).

Stage 3. Corresponds to the haematogenous dissemination of either ACD at a distance (stage 3A) or systemic reactivation of ACD (stage 3B).

Keep in mind that patch testing is the mainstay of etiological diagnosis for all stages of ACDS.

The concept and stages of ACDS are summarized in Fig. 2.2.

2.2.1
Stage 1 of ACDS

By definition, stage 1 of ACDS includes all clinical aspects of ACD at the site(s) of application of contact allergen(s), in terms of morphological aspects and/or localizations.

Morphological Aspects

Morphological aspects of ACD are varied. The commonest are erythematous plaques (with or without oedema) and/or erythemato-vesicular or erythemato-bullous eruptions, evolving sometimes to oozing dermatitis. In a chronic stage, clinical signs of ACD are those of an erythematous, dry and scaly dermatitis.

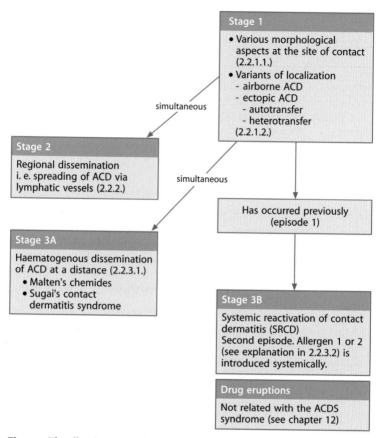

Fig. 2.2. The allergic contact dermatitis syndrome (ACDS): staging by symptomatology

   Clinical variants of ACD are infrequently observed. They are manifold, and can be described as follows:

- Purpuric ACD. This variant is mainly observed on the lower legs and/or feet, and has been reported with a wide variety of allergens (i.e. anti-inflammatory non-steroidal topical drugs, textile dyes, etc.). Purpuric lesions are prominent or associated with eczematous symptoms (sometimes bullous on the lower part of legs and/or feet). They may occur in other regions of the body. Purpura is the clinical manifestation of the extravasation of erythrocytes into dermal tissue and epidermis.

- Lichenoid ACD. Lichenoid ACD is rare. Its clinical features mimic lichen planus (e.g. from metallic dyes in tattoos or from corals). Oral lichenoid ACD looks like oral lichen planus (e.g. from dental amalgams).
- Pigmented ACD. It is mainly described in Oriental populations; it is fully described in Sect. 3.15.
- Lymphomatoid ACD. This variant cannot be defined as a clinical distinctive entity; it is based only on histopathological criteria. Clinical signs (non-diagnostic) are erythemato-oedematous plaques, sometimes very infiltrated, at the site(s) of application of contact allergen(s). Histopathological examination reveals the presence of an important dermal (and sometimes subdermal) infiltrate, displaying features of pseudolymphoma, i.e. mainly lymphohistiocytic with a few neutrophils and/or eosinophils. Immunopathological investigation permits the exclusion of malignant lymphocytic proliferation.

We stress that, in all these variants of ACD, patch testing is equally useful; the clinical signs of positive patch test reactions are eczematous in nature, and therefore identical to those observed in "classic" ACD.

Topographical Variants

ACD can display some topographical peculiarities that may be misleading for every trained dermatologist. This mainly refers to cases of "ectopic" ACD and airborne ACD.

Ectopic dermatitis can follow:

- Autotransfer. A typical example is nail lacquer ACD, located on the eyelids or lateral aspects of the neck (transfer of contact allergen by fingers).
- Heterotransfer. The often-quoted example is transfer of the allergen(s) to the partner. Such events have been described as connubial ACD, or consort ACD, or ACD *per procurationem*; note that in these circumstances, the patient applying the allergen is usually free of any symptoms.

Another pitfall for clinicians is *airborne ACD*. Allergen(s) is (are) transported by air as dust particles, vapours, or gasses. In most cases, ACD involves the face, neck, and/or décolleté. There is usually no spare area, contrary to phototoxic and/or photoallergic contact dermatitis. Limits of eczematous lesions are ill-defined. There is no definite clue to make a clinical distinction between irritant and allergic airborne contact dermatitis. Patch testing is therefore of utmost diagnostic value.

2.2.2
Stage 2 of ACDS

Stage 2 of ACDS is linked with the regional dissemination via lymphatic vessels of ACD from the primary site of application of the allergen(s). In most cases, ACD lesions are more pronounced at the site(s) of application of the allergen(s), and disseminating lesions fade progressively from the primary site. They appear as erythematous or erythemato-vesicular plaques with poorly defined margins. In some other cases, extending lesions are more pronounced than those located at the primary site. This paradoxical observation is not fully understood. It sometimes occurs with, e.g., anti-inflammatory non-steroidal drugs or antibiotics.

Three clinical variants of regional dissemination involve more intricate immunological mechanisms. These include:

a. True *erythema multiforme lesions*, displaying both clinical and histopathological signs of erythema multiforme. Such reactions have been reported with several allergens [5].
b. *Erythema multiforme-like lesions* presenting clinically as "targeted" lesions typical of erythema multiforme, but histopathological signs of a spongiotic dermatitis, characteristic for eczematous dermatitis [5]. The two syndromes (a) and (b) are well documented in some publications, whereas in some others there is no clear-cut distinction between the two, due to a lack of histopathological investigations.
c. An additional variant has been described by Goh [5] under the name of "*urticarial papular and plaque eruption*", a term which is self-explanatory.

In the meantime, widespread secondary lesions can occur simultaneously at a distance from the primary site (stage 3A). In all of these variants, patch testing is of diagnostic value; the clinical signs of positive patch test reactions are similar to those observed in "classic" ACD.

2.2.3
Stage 3 of ACDS

Stage 3 of ACDS includes two distinct entities, leading sometimes to unexpected confusion in the current literature. A clear-cut distinction between the two entities is fully described below.

Stage 3A of ACDS

Stage 3A of ACDS can be defined as a generalized dissemination of skin lesions – via blood vessels from the primary site of application of the allergen. It is considered that the allergen penetrates through normal and/or lesional skin and reaches distant skin sites (haematogenous dissemination) where it provokes secondary (or "ide") reactions. These reactions appear as symmetrical erythematous, sometimes slightly elevated plaques, more rarely vesicular or squamous (Fig. 2.3). They are of "pompholyx-type" on palmar and/or plantar skin.

Malten [6] coined the term "chemides" to describe the various skin manifestations at distant sites. Chemides are always concomitant with ACD lesions at the primary site(s) of application of the allergen.

Malten's historical description was rediscovered by Sugai, under the name of "contact dermatitis syndrome" [7]. Sugai makes a clear distinction between "systemic contact dermatitis syndrome" and "systemic contact-type dermatitis" (see Sect. 2.2.3, stage 3B of ACDS). The sensitization processes and pathways of these two conditions are different: contact dermatitis syndrome (syn: chemides) is provoked by percutaneous absorption of the causative allergen(s) from the primary site of application, whereas in systemic contact-type dermatitis, allergen(s) are introduced by systemic administration (ingestion, inhalation, or injection). The consequence of the latter can be defined as a haematogenous contact-type dermatitis (see Sect. 2.2.3, stage 3B of ACDS).

Sugai added to Malten's initial description some clinical variants, such as true erythema multiforme lesions, erythema multiforme-like lesions, and/or Goh's "urticarial papular and plaque eruption", all types of lesions being similar to those reported in stage 2 of ACDS [8, 9].

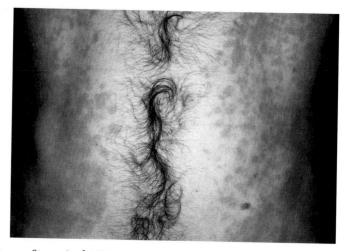

Fig. 2.3. Stage 3A of ACDS. Secondary ("ide") symmetrical reactions at distant skin sites (haematogenous dissemination) from the primar skin site of sensitization to benzocaine

Stages 2 and 3A of ACDS can be present simultaneously in the same individual. The concomitant occurrence of both stages of lesions illustrates the clinical complexity of ACDS.

In stage 3A of ACDS, patch testing remains the milestone of investigation, providing accurate positive reactions, similar to those obtained in stage 2 of ACDS.

Among contact allergens involved in stage 3A of ACDS and reported in the literature, some deserve special interest: paraphenylenediamine, cobalt, nickel, mercury, mercuric chloride, corticosteroids, and nonsteroidal anti-inflammatory agents.

Stage 3B of ACDS

Stage 3B of ACDS has been described many years ago independently as:

■ **Baboon Syndrome** [10]. This term is not satisfactory, since it tends erroneously to circumscribe symptoms to limited skin areas, i.e. buttocks, groin, perineal region; therefore it does not take into account other skin sites, which are involved as well.

■ **Fisher's Systemic Contact Dermatitis.** The term is widely used in dermatology [11]. Nevertheless, it is a misnomer, due to the lack of precise meaning in the definition itself.

In essence, the most appropriate expression could be *systemic reactivation of allergic contact dermatitis* (SRCD) [1]. It considers the chain of events resulting in the occurrence of stage 3B of ACDS.

The following successive steps are:

1. First episode
   A first event of ACD to a well-defined contact allergen (allergen 1) has occurred in the past (weeks or even years before episode 2). All clinical symptoms have vanished completely, when contact with allergen 1 has ceased. Sometimes, patients have forgotten about it; this emphasizes the need for a complete clinical history (a general rule in the field of contact allergy).

2. Second episode
   In some cases, the substance (molecule 1) is introduced systemically (ingestion, inhalation, injection) and its use is followed by a more or less generalized skin rash, usually in a symmetrical pattern (as in Sect. 2.2.3.1, stage 3A of ACDS). The molecule is the true allergen (allergen 1). In other cases, another substance (molecule 2) is used systemically and provokes SRCD. This could be related to two different mechanisms:

a. Molecule 2 is chemically closely related to molecule 1. Both are allergenic and there is cross-sensitization (see Sect. 3.13). Molecule 2 is therefore considered allergen 2.

b. Another possibility is that molecules 1 and 2 are not allergenic as such, but are both transformed into another common molecule, which is the allergen (responsible for episodes 1 and 2).

The clinical signs observed in stage 3B of ACDS share a similar pattern with skin lesions observed in stage 3A of ACDS (Fig. 2.4). The only difference is that in stage 3B, no current skin contact occurs (episode 2).

SRCD is a good indication for patch testing. Positive patch test reactions are diagnostic [12].

There is a clear-cut frontier between stage 3B of ACDS (SRCD) and other immunologically related drug eruptions. In the latter, the allergens have never been applied previously onto the skin; no anterior process of skin sensitization has occurred (absence of episode 1). Patch testing in drug eruptions is discussed at length in Chap. 12.

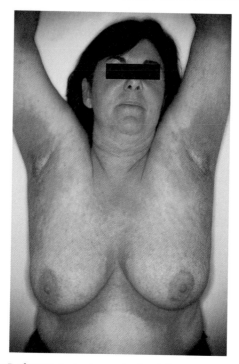

Fig. 2.4. Stage 3B of ACDS. Systemic reactivatin of allergic contact dermatitis provoked by a drug containing aminophylline (theophylline + ethylenediamine) in a patient previously sensitized to ethylenediamine by skin contact

2.3
Other Skin Diseases in Which Patch Testing Is of Major Interest

Patch testing is also highly recommended in patients suffering from various eczematous conditions, considered (partly or entirely) endogenous. The philosophy behind this strategy is related to the fact that in many cases ACD may worsen underlying dermatitis.

Thus, the purpose of patch testing is clearly defined: its results permit further avoidance of contact allergens in the management of eczematous

Table 2.1. Eczematous (endogenous) diseases in which patch testing is recommended

Atopic dermatitis
Nummular dermatitis (nummular eczema)
Seborrhoeic dermatitis (when presenting episodes of acute inflammation)
Asteatotic eczema
Stasis dermatitis
Eczematous lesions around leg ulcers
Pompholyx and/or dyshidrotic eczema (see Sect. 2.5)
Lichenification

conditions. A list of eczematous (endogenous) diseases is presented in Table 2.1.

In our view, accurate patch testing needs to be performed, not only with standard allergens, but also with topical corticosteroids and preservatives. A correct methodology of patch testing (as explained in Chap. 3) is of prime importance.

Psoriatic patients, who have been treated with several topical drugs, may benefit from patch testing. Special attention should be paid to corticosteroids and vitamin D3 analogues (calcipotriol, tacalcitol, calcitriol).

Apart from this, patch testing may be suitable in any other skin condition, whenever the clinician suspects a past or recent history of superimposed ACD.

2.4
An Algorithmic Approach: The Key Role of Patch Testing

Each patient, presenting or having presented with clinical signs suggestive of ACD, requires a complete investigation, built on grounds of evidence-based dermatology. An algorithmic approach of problems is a very efficient way to reach a good evaluation in terms of diagnosis and management ("holistic approach"). The procedure is extremely useful, in particular when dealing with hand dermatitis, a daily challenge for dermatologists. In this perspective, patch testing is one of the pieces of the jigsaw puzzle (see Fig. 2.5). A similar approach can be applied to other situations.

2.5
Hand Dermatitis: Procedures Applied in Differential Diagnosis

Hand dermatitis is a difficult problem, the management of which requires great skill and expertise [14]. Positive and differential diagnosis is crucial. Hand dermatitis may be multifactorial, so that more than one diagnosis has to be kept in mind. The systematic use of an algorithmic approach, including targeted patch testing, is very informative.

2.5.1
Hand Dermatitis: Exogenous and Endogenous Factors

The occurrence of hand dermatitis in a patient may imply exogenous and/or endogenous factors. In each case the balance between these two factors needs precise evaluation (Fig. 2.5) as stressed many years ago by Fregert [13].

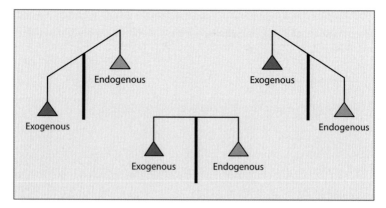

Fig. 2.5. The evaluation of exogenous and endogenous factors in hand dermatitis. (From [15])

2.5.2
A Classification of Hand Dermatitis

The following classification of hand dermatitis is proposed, taking into account the occurrence of exogenous and/or endogenous factors (Table 2.2) [15]. It is obvious that several other dermatoses can affect hands [14]. This classification is willingly limited to the most common situations, being either eczematous or involving differential diagnosis with eczema. Some skin diseases deserve a precise definition.

■ **Tinea Manuum.** Tinea manuum is synonymous with fungal infection of the hands by dermatophytes. The clinical picture on the back of the hands is similar to that observed on other parts of the body, i.e. round-

Table 2.2. Proposal for a classification of hand dermatitis (from [15])

A. Exogenous Irritant contact dermatitis: frictional[a], chemical[a]
Allergic contact dermatitis
Protein contact dermatitis (see Sect. 10.2) and contact urticaria (see Sect. 10.1)
(Tinea manuum)
B. Endogenous Atopic dermatitis (see Chap. 6)
Nummular dermatitis (nummular eczema)
Pompholyx and/or dyshidrotic eczema
Hyperkeratotic palmar dermatitis
Psoriasis
Fingertip dermatitis

[a] In some cases, hand dermatitis is the result of the occurrence of two (or more) combined conditions, e.g. irritant and allergic contact dermatitis, nummular dermatitis and irritant contact dermatitis, etc. Atopic dermatitis can involve both exogenous and/or endogenous factors. Some authors prefer the term "irritant contact dermatitis with an atopic background"; this is misleading, since not only irritants but also contact allergens and proteins can penetrate into the skin and be responsible for clinical manifestations.

shaped erythematosquamous lesions, with an elevated margin, either scaly or vesicular. In contrast, *tinea manuum* of the palms is a whitish scaly dermatosis without any inflammatory component. Skin creases appear as white prominent crossing lines. Erythema is generally absent. Abundant floury material is peeled off easily by curettage. Microscopic investigation is diagnostic.

■ **Nummular Dermatitis.** Nummular dermatitis (nummular eczema) is a variety of eczema of unknown origin. It is claimed that an atopic background does exist in certain cases. Eczematous lesions are round or oval-shaped, either vesicular and oozing, or dry and scaly. The localization on the palms is sometimes described as "apron dermatitis".

■ **Pompholyx.** Pompholyx is defined as a clinical variant of eczematous lesions, involving exclusively palmar skin and/or lateral aspects of the fingers. It is generally accepted that pompholyx is synonymous with dyshidrotic eczema [14]. Clinical symptoms are characterized by the occurrence of numerous vesicles, either isolated or grouped in crops that appear on normal skin or underlying erythema. Itching is often severe. Considered in many cases endogenous (an atopic background has been advocated mainly in children), it can be triggered by several environmental factors, such as tobacco smoking, wet/and or hot work conditions, and hot climate.

Research for etiological factors may be useful. Indeed it has been argued that, in some cases, pompholyx reflects an "ide" reaction to ACD or mycotic infections; in some others, it could be a clinical manifestation of SRCD, in particular to drugs or food ingredients, like spices. A particular relationship between pompholyx and nickel ingestion in nickel-sensitive patients has been advocated [16], but it is still controversial. Oral challenge with nickel is sometimes positive [16].

When pompholyx evolves to a chronic stage, lesions are dry and scaly. At this erythematosquamous stage, differential diagnosis may be difficult with other eczematous conditions or psoriasis.

■ **Hyperkeratotic Palmar Dermatitis.** This condition is characterized by the outcome on the palms of hyperkeratotic sharply demarcated plaques. Deep, painful, sometimes bleeding crevices are common. Erythema is usually very pronounced with well-defined margins, extending around hyperkeratotic plaques, but, in some cases, it is totally absent. Itching, if any, is usually moderate. Mechanical factors can sometimes be implied (hyperkeratotic variant of frictional dermatitis), but, in most cases, environmental factors cannot be traced; therefore hyperkeratotic palmar dermatitis is considered endogenous. This optional view reflects our incomplete understanding of the mechanisms involved in the impaired keratinization of the stratum corneum, in relation or not with an inflammatory process.

■ **Psoriasis.** Psoriasis of the hands is common. Lesions are typical on the back of the hands. Palmar psoriasis is often difficult to diagnose, when not associated with lesions on other skin sites. In some cases, it cannot be differentiated from hyperkeratotic palmar dermatitis, with which it shares common features. Biopsy is of no help. Nail examination is important, since psoriatic nail lesions are diagnostic.

■ **Fingertip Dermatitis.** Chapping of the fingertips is a common event. Painful crevices and bleeding do occur in severe cases. We have stressed [15] that fingertip dermatitis limited to the thumb, index (and eventually medius) of one or both hands frequently implies irritant (frictional and/or chemical) or allergenic factors. In those cases, fingertip dermatitis may be typical of (a) irritant contact dermatitis, (b) allergic contact dermatitis, or (c) protein contact dermatitis. We have coined the term "gripping form" of fingertip dermatitis [15]. Such considerations are far too simple; in many of these cases the skin condition remains unclear and it is therefore considered endogenous, environmental factors playing only an adverse role. When some fingers are randomly involved, whereas others are spared, or in case of complete involvement of all fingers of both hands, etiology is even more obscure.

2.5.3
Tools of Investigation

Several procedures are available in the diagnostic approach of hand dermatitis. They are listed in Table 2.3.

Table 2.3. Hand dermatitis: Tools of investigation[a]

Accurate clinical history, obtained by questionnaire
Careful clinical examination
Patch testing
Prick testing
Microscopic examination of scales collected by curettage (in search of dermatophytes)
IgE blood level (of minor interest, to find an atopic background)

[a] Skin biopsy provides questionable results in most cases.

2.5.4
Hand Dermatitis: Some Examples of an Algorithmic Approach

Two examples of an algorithmic approach applied to the diagnosis of hand dermatitis are presented in Figs. 2.6 and 2.7.

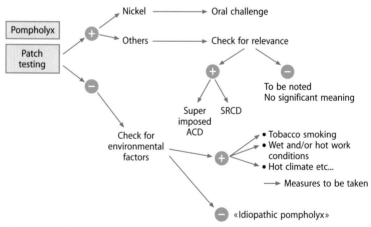

Fig. 2.6. An algorithmic approach to pompholyx

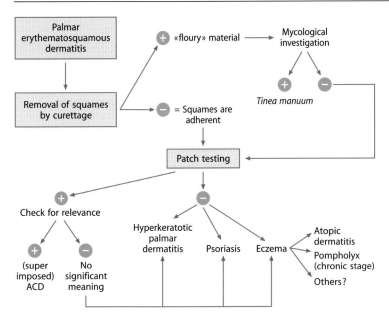

Fig. 2.7. An algorithmic approach to palmar erythematosquamous dermatitis

References

1. Lachapelle JM (2001) Dermato-allergologie de contact. Nouv Dermatol (Strasbourg) 20:450–452
2. The American Heritage Dictionary (1985) Second college edition. Houghton Mifflin Company, Boston
3. van der Valk PGM, Maibach HI (1995) The irritant contact dermatitis syndrome. CRC Press, Boca Raton
4. Maibach HI, Johnson HL (1975) Contact urticaria syndrome. Contact urticaria to diethyltoluamide (immediate type hypersensitivity). Arch Dermatol 111:726–730
5. Goh CL (2001) Non eczematous contact reactions. In: Rycroft RJG, Menné T, Frosch P, Lepoittevin JP (eds) Textbook of contact dermatitis, 3rd edn. Springer, Berlin, pp 413–431
6. Malten KE, Nater JP, van Ketel WG (1976) Patch testing guidelines. Dekker and van de Vegt, Nijmegen
7. Sugai T (1988) Contact dermatitis syndrome and unusual skin manifestations. Skin Research 30:8–17

8. Sugai T (2000) Contact dermatitis syndrome (CDS) Environ Dermatol (Nagoya) 7:543–544
9. Kato Y, Sugiura M, Hashimoto R, Ogawa H, Hayakawa R (2001) Eight cases of contact dermatitis syndrome. Environ Dermatol (Nagaya) 8:41–47
10. Andersen KE, Hjorth N, Menné T (1984) The baboon syndrome: systemically induced allergic contact dermatitis. Contact Dermatitis 10:97–101
11. Fisher AA (1986) Systemic contact-type dermatitis. In: Contact dermatitis. Lea and Febiger, Philadelphia, pp 119–131
12. Menné T, Veien K (2001) Systemic contact dermatitis. In: Rycroft RJG, Menné T, Frosch P, Lepoittevin JP (eds) Textbook of contact dermatitis, 3rd edn. Springer, Berlin, pp 355–366
13. Fregert S (1981) Manual of contact dermatitis, 2nd edn. Munksgaard, Copenhagen
14. Menné T, Maibach HI (2000) Hand eczema, 2nd edn. CRC Press, Boca Raton
15. Lachapelle JM (2001) Les dermatites des mains: approche algorithmique des onze diagnostics différentiels de base. In: Lachapelle JM, Tennstedt D (eds) Progrès en Dermato-Allergologie, Bruxelles, 2001. John Libbey Eurotext, Montrouge (France) pp 1–10
16. Veien NK, Menné T (1990) Nickel contact allergy and a nickel-restricted diet. Semin Dermatol 9:197

CHAPTER 3

The Methodology of Patch Testing

J.-M. LACHAPELLE , H. I. MAIBACH

3.1
Historical Background

Jozef Jadassohn is universally acknowledged as the father of patch testing [1]. At the time of his discovery in 1895, he was Professor of Dermatology at Breslau University (now Wroclaw in Poland). He initially reported a patient who had developed an eczematous reaction to mercury plasters. He recognized the potential for eczematous reactions to occur in some (sensitized) patients, when chemicals were applied to their skin; he thereby introduced the world to the contact test, then referred to as "Funktionelle Hautprüfung" [2].

Bruno Bloch (Professor at Basel and Zurich Universities) is considered by the international community as one of the more outstanding pioneers in the field of patch testing, continuing and expanding Jadassohn's clinical and experimental work. In some textbooks and papers, patch testing is sometimes quoted as the Jadassohn-Bloch technique.

In retrospect, it is difficult to assess the real place of the patch test procedure for the diagnosis of contact dermatitis between 1895 and the 1960s. Some points seem obvious:

1. The technique was used extensively in some European clinics, and ignored in others.
2. No consensus was reached concerning material, concentrations of allergens, time of reading, reading scores, etc.
3. Differential diagnosis between irritant *versus* allergic contact dermatitis was often unclear.

It is no exaggeration to say that patch testers were acting like skilled craftsmen. Nevertheless they provided, step by step, new information on contact dermatitis.

During that long period, clinicians often equated a positive patch test with the fulfilment of Koch's postulate [3]. They inferred that because a patient with dermatitis was shown to develop a positive reaction to compound X, the same compound must therefore be the cause of the dermatitis. In other words, there was little attempt to interpret correctly patch test results. Relevance was a neglected concept.

Credit must be given to the former members of the International Contact Dermatitis Research Group (ICDRG) for their invaluable contribution to the standardization and interpretation of patch test procedures. Their efforts have encouraged many dermatologists, immunologists, chemists and pharmacists.

Patch testing is now a well-recognized diagnostic tool, constantly being refined.

3.2
Definition and Aims

Patch testing aims to reproduce "in miniature" an eczematous reaction, by applying allergens under occlusion on intact skin of patients suspected to be allergic. It is the in vivo visualization of the elicitation phase of a delayed-type hypersensitivity (type IV) reaction.

Patch testing is not intended to reflect an irritant reaction, considering its occurrence an untoward event, to be avoided by any means.

"Patch test reactions properly performed and interpreted are acceptable as scientific proof of a state of allergic sensitization" [4].

A perfect patch test should give no false-positive nor false-negative reactions. Furthermore, the ideal patch test should cause as few adverse reactions as possible, particularly no patch test sensitization. False-positive, false-negative and adverse reactions are all dose-dependent.

Patch testing is submitted to general rules of evidence-based medicine applied to investigative procedures.

A good screening test for a given disease in a given population must meet several requirements. In addition to simplicity, safety and low cost, it must have a very good *positive predictive value* (percentage of true cases in those with a positive test, when this test is used in a given population) and good *negative predictive value* (percentage of disease-free individuals in those with a negative test, when this test is used in a given population).

Positive and negative predictive values depend not only on *sensitivity* (probability of a positive test in an individual with the disease) and *specificity* (probability of a negative test in an individual without the disease), but also on the prevalence of the disease in the given population. A good screening test must also be reliable, which means that it has to be precise and have good *intraobserver and interobserver reproducibility* [5].

Conventional patch testing, as described in this chapter, is used worldwide. Allergens are produced and purchased separately from patch test units plus tapes.

True Test is an alternative way of patch testing described in Chap. 9.

3.3
Patch Test Units

Earlier (non-chamber) patch tests, such as Leukotest, Porotest, Neo-Dermotest, and others have been withdrawn from the market, except one: Curatest F.

Curatest F is a non-chamber patch test unit consisting of adhesive strips for patch tests made of transparent film hypoallergenic adhesive, 10 test discs per strip. It is not of common use nowadays.

Curatest F is marketed by Lohmann GmbH & Co. KG, Postfach 23 43, 56513 Neuwied, Germany.

3.3.1
Finn Chamber

Finn Chamber is a round aluminium patch test device which provides good occlusion because of the chamber design [6]. The 8-mm inner diameter provides a 50-mm² area and about 20 µl volume. The outer diameter is 11 mm, and the distance between the chambers is 20 mm. Finn Chambers are available mounted on an acrylate-based adhesive tape, Scanpor Alpharma AS, Norgesplaster Facility, Kristiansand, Norway.

Finn Chambers on Scanpor (Fig. 3.1) are available in strips of 10 (2 × 5) and 1 chamber(s). The strips of 10 chambers are practical when testing with a large number of substances, e.g. with routine tests. Smaller strips are suitable for small test series and individual tests.

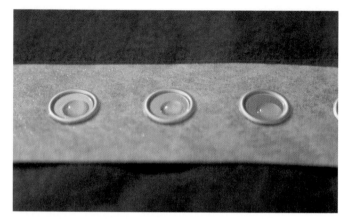

Fig. 3.1. Finn Chambers filled with allergens dispersed in petrolatum

Most commercial test substances are suitable for Finn Chambers. The substances incorporated in petrolatum are applied directly into the chamber. For liquids (e.g. formaldehyde), a filter paper disc in placed in the chamber and saturated with the liquid.

Finn Chambers may be safely used for patch testing mercurials if these are dispersed in petrolatum [7], but are unsuitable for aqueous solutions of some mercurials, due to a complete corrosion of the aluminium chamber [7]. Polypropylene-coated chambers (thus avoiding corrosion) are available on request.

The Finn Chamber Tray keeps the test strips in good order when applying the test substances. The trays are stackable, which saves space on the work surface. When removing the tests, the occlusion is verified by a ring-shaped depression around each test.

For locating the test sites, a special device, Reading Plate is recommended. Reading Plate can also be used when removing the tests (Fig. 3.2).

Apart from standard 8-mm (inner diameter) Finn Chambers, large 12-mm (inner diameter) Finn Chambers can be purchased (200 strips of 1 chamber). These are of special interest when using the Atopy Patch Test (see Sect. 6.2). Extra-large 18-mm (inner diameter) Finn Chambers are intended to be used only for special experimental purposes.

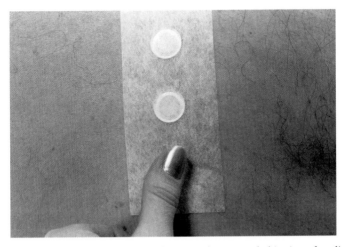

Fig. 3.2. Finn Chambers: mode of application. After removal, skin sites of application can be checked by the Finn Chamber Reading Plate

The methodology of use of Finn Chambers is as follows:

a. Lay out, with backing removed, all of the chambers to be used.
b. Start with n°1 of the standard tray, apply a small amount of allergen to each disk. A 5-mm ribbon of petrolatum-based allergen is sufficient. Proceed in sequence through the trays to be tested.
c. For liquid allergens, place a filter paper disk in the chamber, and apply one drop of liquid, just sufficient to soak the disk. Petrolatum patches can be made up a few hours in advance; liquid patches should be made up at the last minute.

When all patches in a Finn Chamber patch test show red infiltrated papular rings, contact sensitivity to aluminium should be suspected [8], but it can be considered exceptional.

Finn Chamber is marketed by Epitest Ltd Oy, Rannankoukku 22, 04300 Tuusula, Finland (Tel.: +358-9-2755366, Fax: +358-9-2754335, e-mail: epitest@epitest.fi).

3.3.2
Plastic Square Chambers

Several companies have recently introduced different models of square plastic chambers as an alternative. The square shape of the chambers is intended theoretically to differentiate allergic and irritant reactions.

IQ Square Chamber Chemotechnique

The IQ Chamber Chemotechnique is made of additive-free polyethylene plastic. Undesired sides effects in the form of allergic reactions to the test unit itself are avoided due to the chemical stability of the polyethylene plastic.

The IQ chambers are supplied in units of 10 square chambers (in two rows of five chambers/row) on a hypoallergenic acrylic-based non-woven adhesive tape, providing good occlusion and fixation of the test unit to the skin (Fig. 3.3). The tape with the chambers is protected by a stiff plastic cover, with ten compartments that correspond to the chambers on the tape.

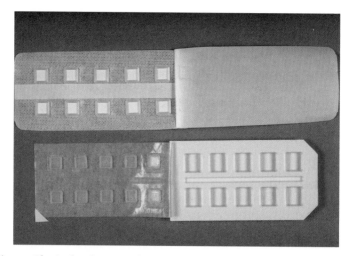

Fig. 3.3. Plastic chambers: van der Bend Square Chamber (up); IQ Square Chamber Chemotechnique (down)

The volume of the chamber is 65 µl, and the inside area of the chamber is 9 × 9 mm (81 mm^2). The bottom of the chamber is filled with filter paper. The distance between the chambers is 12 mm in the row and 20 mm between the rows. The width of the tape is 68 mm, and the length is 142 mm.

IQ Chambers are delivered in two sizes of cardboard boxes containing either 100 units or 50 units per box.

The IQ Chamber is marketed by Chemotechnique Diagnostics, P.O. Box 80, Edvard Ols Väg 2, 23042 Tygelsjö, Malmö, Sweden (Tel.: +46-40-466077, Fax: +46-40-466700, e-mail: info@chemotechnique.se)

van der Bend Square Chamber

The van der Bend Square Chamber is made of an additive-free polymer. Undesired side effects in the form of allergic reactions to the test unit itself are avoided due to the chemical stability of the polymer.

van der Bend Chambers can be delivered already fixed on tape but also joined in a row without tape, which makes it easy to apply the test on a porous adhesive (e.g. Fixomull Beiersdorf) that can be chosen by the dermatologist carrying out the test.

The volume of the chamber is 100 ml, and the inside area of the chamber is 10 × 10 mm (100 mm^2). The distance between the chambers is 15 mm.

There is a standard Whatman filter paper 1 × 1 cm, mechanically fixed without glue in each chamber (Fig. 3.3).

The van der Bend Square Chamber is marketed by van der Bend B.V., Postbus 73, 3230 AB Brielle, The Netherlands (Tel.: +31-18-1018055, Fax: +31-18-1017450).

Haye's Test Square Chamber

The Haye's Test Square Chamber is made of a white speenlaced hydrophilic unbleached non-woven polyester, devoid of any allergenic properties. The chambers are supplied in units of 10 square chambers (in two rows of five chambers/row), on a hypoallergenic solventless acrylic adhesive (MED5761U). The tape with the chambers is protected by a transparent protection cover.

The volume of the chamber is 40 µl, and the inside area of the chamber is 8 × 8 mm (64 mm^2). The bottom of the chamber is filled with Whatman filter paper, 0.6 cm², fixed without adhesive. The distance between the chambers is 9 mm in the row and 23 mm between the rows. The width of the tape is 70 mm, and the length is 120 mm. Chambers are delivered in a box containing 100 units.

For use with Haye's Test Chambers (when kept in the refrigerator), Haye's Test Chambers Sealings were developed (designed covers). They are made of environmentally responsible synthetic material and cover all 10 test chambers of the plaster without having to remove the Kraft release liner beforehand. Haye's Test Chambers Sealings are delivered in boxes containing 60 pieces.

The Haye's Test Square Chamber is marketed by HAL Allergenen Lab. B.V., Parklaan 125, 2011 KT Haarlem, The Netherlands (Tel.: +31-23-5319512, Fax: +31-23-5322418, e-mail: sales@hal-allergic.nl).

3.3.3
Reinforcement of Patch Test Units

The patch test units may be reinforced by extra tape, stuck at the margins or covering the total surface of the original tape and extending over its margins. The procedure is particularly recommended in hot climate, to avoid detachment of the strips. Its use is also advisable but facultative in temperate climate.

Fixomull stretch Beiersdorf (10 m × 15 cm rolls) is convenient for this purpose.

3.4
A General Overview of Allergens

3.4.1
Allergens

The standard and/or additional series of patch test allergens are sold by two companies, working in close connection with the ICDRG and other international and/or national groups.

- Trolab Hermal, 21462, Reinbek, Germany (Tel.: +49-40-72704266, Fax: +49-40-72704317, e-mail: info@hermal.de)

- Chemotechnique Diagnostics, P.O. Box 80 Edvard Ols väg 2, 23042 Tygelsjö, Malmö, Sweden (Tel.: +46-40-466077, Fax: +46-40-466700, e-mail: info@chemotechnique.se)

According to those suppliers' product catalogues, the allergens can be considered chemically defined and pure. The substances with a petrolatum vehicle are supplied in 5-ml propylpropylene syringes, while those in a liquid solution are supplied in 10-ml polypropylene dropper bottles. The vast majority of allergens of the standard and/or additional series are dispersed in white petrolatum (Fig. 3.4). The petrolatum used as a vehicle is Penreco Snow White, considered to be the purest on the market [9].

White petrolatum can be considered inert when applied onto the skin, but may be responsible in exceptional cases for an irritant reaction.

A few allergens cannot be dispersed in petrolatum, due to their chemical instability. It is the reason why they are supplied in aqueous solutions. Some examples include formaldehyde, Cl+Me-isothiazolinone, phenylmercuric acetate, coco-amidopropylbetaine, ammonium thioglycolate, chlorhexidine digluconate, benzalkonium chloride, etc. Hydrocortisone-

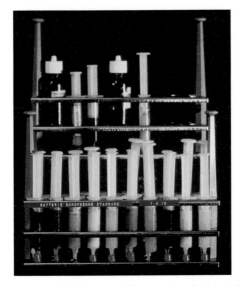

Fig. 3.4. Tray with contact allergens (standard series)

17-butyrate is dissolved in ethanol 70%. A extensive list of chemicals not available in marketed lists of allergens is given in de Groot's textbook [10]. This provides useful and accurate information about test concentrations and vehicles. The vehicles which are referred are water, acetone, ethanol 70%, methylethylketone, olive oil and petrolatum. Liquid vehicles are recommended for some allergens, since they facilitate penetration into the skin, but they have also some drawbacks. Solvents may evaporate, which does not favour exact dosing, and most test solutions must be freshly prepared. Liquid vehicles are used mainly when testing chemicals and products brought by patients, and in research projects.

In textbooks on contact dermatitis and patch testing, and in suppliers' catalogues, the concentration of an allergen is given as a percentage. In one catalogue [11], molality (m) is given together with percentage (weight/weight). The traditional method of presenting concentrations as a percentage is simple and probably practical, but has been questioned [12], as we do not know if this means weight/weight, volume/volume, volume/weight, or weight/volume. Especially when comparing substances and in research projects, it is the number of moles applied that is of interest.

Finding the ideal test concentration is complicated; the currently recommended concentrations have been determined taking many important factors into account.

The general principle has always been to use the highest concentration which does not provoke any irritation, when testing in groups of patients enrolled in prospective joint studies. Doing so, false-positive (irritant) and false-negative (due to a too-low concentration) reactions are avoided. Therefore, the choice of the concentration tends to reach an ideal (but sometimes unattainable) compromise.

The allergens should be kept in a cool dark place (refrigerator) to minimize degradation. In accordance with their stability, it is recommended that all substances should be renewed according to the expiry stated on the labels of the allergens. Non-marketed allergens are prepared fresh; allergens diluted in liquids should be kept in dark bottles.

3.4.2
Bioavailability of Allergens

To obtain optimal bioavailability of an allergen, one can influence the following five parameters:

- Intrinsic penetration capacity
- Concentration
- Vehicle
- Occlusivity of patch test system and tape
- Exposure time

Since it is desirable to remove all test strips at the same time, usually at day 2 (48 h), four factors remain and can be varied and optimized by the manufacturers of patch test materials and allergen preparations and by the dermatologist responsible for the testing.

3.4.3
Quality Control of Allergens

The dermatologist is recommended to obtain protocols of chemical analyses and data on purity from suppliers of test preparations.

3.5
Specific Recommendations when Considering Patch Testing Patients

Some general rules as well as recommendations have to be taken into consideration when patch testing patients. This seems useful in practice.

3.5.1
Patch Testing on Intact Skin Is Imperious

The general rule is to avoid by any means patch testing at skin sites presenting currently or recently any type of dermatitis, to avoid false-positive reactions and/or the angry back syndrome (see Sect. 3.14.2). This includes not only contact dermatitis (either primary or "id" reaction) but also atopic dermatitis, nummular eczema and seborrhoeic dermatitis. Similar considerations are applied to various skin diseases, such as pityriasis versicolor, psoriasis, lichen planus, pityriasis rubra pilaris, pityriasis lichenoides, pityriasis rosea and others. Complete healing or remission is needed before patch testing.

3.5.2
Medicaments and Patch Testing

Corticosteroids

Treatment of test sites with topical corticosteroids [13] can give rise to false-negative reactions.

Testing a patient on oral corticosteroids always creates uncertainty. The problem was studied 25–30 years ago [14] by comparing the intensity of test reactions before and during treatment with corticosteroids (20–40 mg prednisone). Diminution and disappearance of test reactions were noted in several cases, but not regularly. These findings have been interpreted as allowing us to test patients on oral doses equivalent to 20 mg of prednisone without missing any important allergies. However, the test reactions studied were strong (+++), and fairly questionable reactions were not evaluated. We conclude that interpretation of patch test results in patients treated with corticosteroids needs great caution; repeating patch testing after treatment discontinuation can be useful when in doubt.

Antihistamines

The interference of antihistamines on patch test results has not been evaluated according to the current rules of evidence-based dermatology. It is generally accepted that antihistamines cannot reduce significantly the intensity of positive patch test reactions; therefore, in most clinics, they are not discontinued when patch testing patients. This rule does not apply to the atopy patch test in atopics (see Chap. 6).

Immunomodulators

There is thus far no comparison of test reactions in allergic patients before and during treatment with oral cyclosporine. It is our experience that cyclosporine (at a dose of 3 mg/kg/day) does not alter the positive answer to potassium dichromate in cement workers suffering from cement allergic contact dermatitis of the hands, but this is considered a very limited experience.

No information exists regarding the influence of azathioprine and cytostatic agents on patch test results.

At present, caution is needed as regards the current use of the new topical immunomodulators tacrolimus and pimecrolimus, since it has been demonstrated that they are efficient in treating atopic dermatitis.

Irradiation

Irradiation with UVB [15] and Grenz rays [16] reduced the number of Langerhans' cells and the intensity of patch test reactions in humans. Repeated suberythema doses of UVB depressed reactivity even at sites shielded during the exposures. This indicates a systemic effect of UVB [15].

From a practical point of view, avoid patch testing on markedly tanned persons, and a minimum of 4 weeks after heavy sun exposure should be allowed before testing.

3.5.3
Pregnancy and Patch Testing

There are no indications that the minute amounts of allergens absorbed in patch testing could influence the fetus, but in cases of miscarriage or deformity it is natural to blame several things, including medical investigations. Therefore, the general rule adopted by the members of the ICDRG is: do not test pregnant women, taking into account medico-legal considerations, not scientific ones. In some clinics, this view is also adopted for lactating women.

3.5.4
Patch Testing in Children

In children, patch testing has the same indications as in adults. Most authors agree that patch testing in children is safe, the only problems being mainly technical because of the small patch test surface [17]. It is usually advised to use the Finn Chamber. Reinforcement of patch test units is suitable, due to hypermobility of children, which may result in loss of patch test materials.

Instructions should be given to parents about the test procedure and the measures that may be taken to optimize the patch test conditions [17].

There has been much debate about the concentrations of allergens to be used in children. Some authors have recommended lower concentrations, but nowadays, there is a general consensus of using the same concentrations as in adults. Similarly, most authors agree upon the fact of applying in children the classical standard series, as well as additional series, if needed [17]. Some authors have advocated the use of a limited series of patch tests [18] but there is no general agreement about this opinion.

3.6
Application of Patch Tests on the Skin: Some Practical Suggestions

The accurate application of patch test units onto the skin is a prerequisite to ensure optimal reading and interpretation of patch test results.

Some suggestions to optimize the technique of application are listed below:

3.6.1
Test Sites

The preferred site is the upper back (Fig. 3.5). For a small number of allergens, for example at retesting, the outer aspect of the upper arm is also acceptable. False-negative results can be obtained when testing on the lower back or on the volar forearms.

The avoidance of applying patch tests on naevi or seborrhoeic keratoses is self-evident, but not always respected.

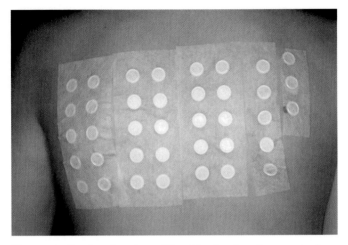

Fig. 3.5. Application of patch test (Finn Chambers) on the upper back

3.6.2
Removal of Hair

On hairy areas of the back it is difficult to get acceptable skin contact, and for this reason clipping is recommended. However, a combination of clipping, petrolatum and tapes sometimes contributes to the irritation seen, which makes reading somewhat difficult. It is advisable to clip hair one or two days before patch testing, whenever possible.

3.6.3
Degreasing of Test Site

In cases of oily skin, gentle treatment with ethanol or other mild solvents could be recommended. The solvent must evaporate before the test strips are applied. Practically, no degreasing is performed in most European clinics.

3.6.4
Application of Test Strips

Test strips should be applied from below with mild pressure to remove air pouches, followed by some moderate strokes with the back of the hand to improve adhesion [19].

3.6.5
Instructions to Patients

Patients should be informed as to the aim of the test; about avoidance of showers, wetting the test site, irradiation and excessive exercise, and about symptoms such as itch and loosening of patches. Written instructions and guidelines for patients are highly recommendable.

3.7
Reading Time

The reading is the most important step in the patch test procedure. It should be done by the clinician him or herself, and interpreted very carefully. There is a need for constructive dialogue between clinician and patient. This requires time, skill and perseverance to achieve the specific aim of tracing the source of allergy. The reading allows the technician to complete past and current history in each individual patient. It cannot be dissociated from the search for relevance or non-relevance (see Chap. 8). A decision must made about whether to continue the investigation by additional patch tests and/or other tests such as repeated open application test (ROAT), for instance (see Sect. 7.4). Therefore, it may be considered that in many cases the reading is only an intermediate step in the investigatory process.

There are controversies in the literature regarding the optimal reading time, as discussed in the following sections. Therefore, the "best" reading time is always a matter of compromise.

3.7.1
Standard Patch Test Occlusion and Reading Time

The standard patch test technique involves application of the test allergen strips on the skin under occlusion for 2 days (48 h). Conventionally patch test reading is performed 15–30 min after the removal of the occlusive strips to allow the transient erythema caused by the occlusive effects of allergens and plasters to subside [20]. This will eliminate false-positive reactions. The 2-day occlusion ensures that adequate allergen penetration has occurred to provoke an allergic contact reaction on the test site.

Reading is further performed at day 3, 4, and/or 7 after occlusion (i.e. 1, 2, 5 days after the removal of the patch test strips) thereafter.

3.7.2
Conventional Patch Test Reading Time

Conventionally, patch test reading is carried out in most patch test clinics at day 2 when the patch test strips are removed, and again at day 4. Allergic reactions are then identified and checked for relevance. Patients are then instructed to report back to the dermatologist should any additional positive reaction appear at day 5 or beyond to detect any late reactors or sensitization that may have occurred.

3.7.3
Reading at Day 2, Day 3, Day 4

Positive reactions at day 2 after the removal of the test strips should not be considered positive unless the reactions persist into day 3 and beyond [21]. True allergic reactions should persist or appear at days 3 and 4.

3.7.4
Reading at Day 7

Reactions occurring at day 7 or later are regarded as late reactions. Some allergens are "late reactors," and delayed positive reactions may appear at day 5 or later. Examples of such late reactors include neomycin and corti-costeroids [22]. In some cases late reactions reflect active sensitization (see Sect. 3.14.1).

3.7.5
Single Reading Versus Multiple Reading

A single reading carried out at day 2 may result in false-negative reactions. Reading of diagnostic patch test should not cease at day 2, as numerous allergic reactions need more time to evolve to become positive. Further recommended reading times include day 3, day 4, and day 7. In most patch test clinics around the world, patch test reading is carried out at day 4.

3.7.6
Day 3 Versus Day 4 Reading

Recent studies have indicated that day 4 reading yields better results (few-er false-negative results) than day 3 reading alone, because some positive results appear only after day 3 [23].

At this stage, it must be recalled that several exogenous factors, e.g. surface concentration of the allergen, total amount applied, penetration properties of the allergens and the vehicle, patch test technique and aller-gen exposure time are major determinants in the elicitation of positive patch test reactions [24].

3.7.7
One-Day Occlusion Versus Two-Day Occlusion

Most authors advocate an exposure time of 48 h. A few comparisons of 1-day (24 h) and 2-day (48 h) allergen exposure show some reactions pos-itive only at day 1 (24 h) and some positive only at day 2 (48 h). A 1-day ex-posure would reduce the number of questionable reactions. No definite conclusion can be drawn from the studies published to date [25].

In tropical climates where the environmental temperature and hu-midity are high, 1-day occlusion may be adequate to elicit positive patch test reactions. The shorter occlusion will be more tolerable to the patients and is more likely to improve compliance and co-operation from patients to accept the patch test procedure [26].

3.7.8
Marking the Skin

When several readings are carried out, it is extremely useful to "mark" the patch test sites.

The Chemotechnique Skin Marker is a special marker designed for efficiently marking the patch test sites. Its content is: methylrosanilin (gentian violet), 1%; silver nitrate, 10%; denatured ethanol/aqua in equal parts ad 100%. The duration of the marking is approximately 5–7 days. Marking may be repeated to ensure durable staining.

For dark skin types or when a non-staining ink is required, the Chemotechnique UV Skin Marker (yellow fluorescent ink) provides a good alternative. Its content is: disulphonic acid derivate of stilbene, 2%; dimethylsulphoxide (DMSO)/denatured ethanol in equal parts ad 100%.

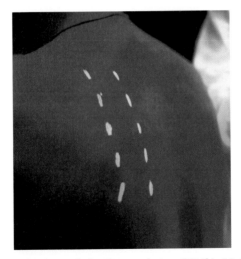

Fig. 3.6. Marking the skin with the Chemotechnique UV Skin Marker: examination under Woods's light

DMSO increases fixation of the ink to the outer layer of the skin. The tip has tapered edges, which facilitates precise markings. The duration of the marking is approximately 5–7 days. The UV Skin Marker requires the use of a Wood's light at each reading session (Fig. 3.6).

Some authors do not use skin markers, but rather a reading plate (i.e. Reading Plate for Finn Chambers on Scanpor Epitest), which is a real template for the patch skin sites (Fig. 3.2).

A practical, clean, durable and inexpensive alternative method of marking was reported recently [27]. It requires A4 (21 × 29.7 cm) transparencies used for transparent photocopies, and two or three colours of dry erasable pens. Contours of patch test areas are carefully marked with a pen. The transparency is used for further readings.

3.7.9
Immediate Urticarial Reactions to Some Allergens

Seldom, some allergens (e.g. balsam of Peru, cinnamic aldehyde) are responsible for an immediate urticarial reaction about 20–30 min after applying patch tests. It is the reason why some authors remove the tests for a short while at 30 min and reapply them immediately at the same site. This practice, that is in essence wise, is not usually carried out by dermatologists. The reaction can be reproduced when applying the allergen in an open test. Meticulous investigators apply systematically in each patient balsam of Peru on the volar aspect of the left forearm, and cinnamic aldehyde on the volar aspect of the right forearm, as a open test (see Sect. 7.2). Readings occur at 20 and 30 min.

3.8
Reading and Scoring Patch Test Results

3.8.1
Nomenclature: Scoring Codes

It is most important for patch tests to be scored according to the reaction seen and not only according to the interpretation placed on the reaction by the reader (Fig. 3.7). Irritant reactions should be recorded as positive

Table 3.1. Scoring of patch test reactions according to Wilkinson et al. [28]

Score	Interpretation
–	Negative
?+	Doubtful reaction[a]
+	Weak (non-vesicular) reaction[b]
++	Strong (oedematous or vesicular) reaction
+++	Extreme (bullous or ulcerative)[c]
NT	Not tested
IR	Irritant reaction of different types

[a] ?+ is a questionable faint or macular (non-palpable) erythema and is not interpreted as proven allergic reaction.
[b] + is a palpable erythema, suggestive of a slight oedematous reaction.
[c] From coalescing vesicles.
Note that photopatch tests (see Chap. 5, Sects. 5.4, 5.5) are graded similarly with a prefix Ph: Ph–, Ph?+, Ph+, Ph++, Ph+++, Ph NT, Ph IR.

irritant and not as negative. In our view, the best scoring system remains that recommended by Wilkinson et al. [28] and reproduced in Table 3.1. Some variants of scoring do exist in textbooks of contact dermatitis; they include the occasional occurrence of papules, as an additional clinical sign of + and ++ reactions. Papules are purposely omitted in our scoring system for two reasons: they do not provide any complementary useful information, and histopathological examination of papules observed in some positive patch test reactions reveals that they are in fact tiny vesicles [29].

Reading and scoring have to be repeated at each individual visit, to check the progression or regression of the reaction (day 2, day 4, day 6 or 7).

3.8.2
Some Remarks About Reading and Scoring

Size of the Reaction

The size of the reaction is different from case to case. The use of current patch test units (i.e. chambers) has limited the size of the reaction to the patch area in most cases; nevertheless, the reaction may sometimes spread

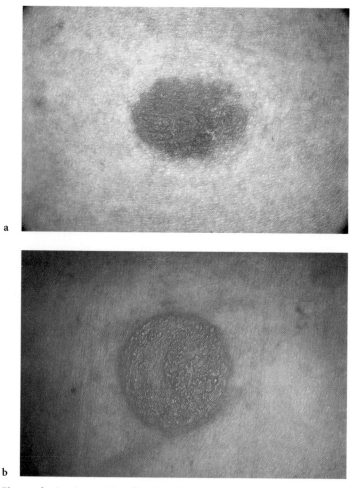

a

b

Fig. 3.7a, b. Scoring positive allergic patch test reactions. **a** + reaction; **b** ++ reaction

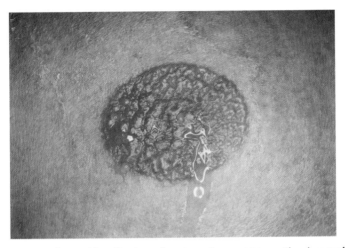

Fig. 3.7c. Scoring positive allergic patch test reactions. **c** +++ reaction (see explanations in text)

all around the patch area, outside of the chamber's margins. It can be concluded that the reactions are more limited nowadays (thus more comfortable for the patient) than previously, when older patch tests (i.e. non-chamber) units were used. Readings are therefore easier, due to the absence of overlap between neighbouring positive reactions.

Edge Effect

The occurrence of "ring-shaped" allergic positive patch test reactions to allergens dissolved in a liquid vehicle (i.e. formaldehyde) is not uncommon [30]. Such reactions can be explained by the accumulation of the chemicals at the periphery of the patch test site. We previously coined the term "edge effect," because some patch test units are square in shape [31]. When using such units, the liquids accumulate at the "edges" of the squares. The occurrence of the "edge" or "ring" effect could be due to pressure. Besides this pressure mechanism, capillary migration could be responsible for an enhanced edge effect. Exceptionally, "ring-shaped" reactions can occur with allergens dispersed in petrolatum, the explanation of which could also be the effect of pressure.

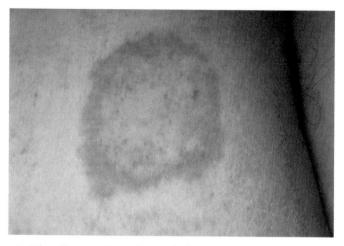

Fig. 3.8. Edge effect: positive patch test to hydrocortisone (see explanations in text)

A particular type of edge effect (Fig. 3.8) can be seen when patch testing with corticosteroids [32]. The margins of the positive test are red, whereas the central area is whitish. This could be related to the vasoconstrictive effect of the corticosteroid, due to an enhanced penetration of the chemicals in the central area. Vasoconstriction and reduction of the inflammatory process most probably counteract the expression of the allergic response.

What Must Be Done in Case of "? +" (Doubtful/Questionable) Reactions?

"? +" reactions are labelled "doubtful" in the files. There is no real problem when allergens of the standard and/or additional series are concerned, since that type of reaction reflects in most cases the true allergic nature of the reaction.

More attention must be paid if the reading occurs in a hot climate, due to the potentially increased irritancy of some allergens, such as the fragrance mix.

A caveat does exist: "? +" reactions cannot be easily interpreted as irritant or allergic when patch testing with less common allergens, and even more so with products of unknown content, the irritancy of which is to a large extent unknown.

In order to circumvent these difficulties, the following strategy can be adopted by the clinician:

a. Repeat the patch test in the patient to check its reproducibility. This may include serial dilutions of the suspected allergen (dose/concentration relationship).
b. Apply the same test in control subjects.
c. Conduct additional investigations in the patient, such as open tests, repeated open application tests (ROATs), and eventually use tests.

To strengthen the validity of such investigations, it should be noted that, when applying patch tests in the same patients (left *versus* right sides of the back), most discrepancies in patch test readings do occur with "? +" and/or "+" reactions [33].

What Must Be Done in Cases of Pustular Reactions?

The occurrence of pustules in positive allergic patch test reactions is not uncommon. This is particularly true with metallic salts (chromate, nickel, cobalt, etc.) mainly, but not exclusively, in atopics. If some doubt does exist in relation with its allergic meaning, repeating the tests would be wise, including a serial dilution test. This step-by-step procedure can avoid false-positive reactions and permits an unequivocal positive or negative reassessment of the allergic nature of the test.

3.9
Irritant Patch Test Reactions

In older days, when patch testing did not respond to definite rules (due to the lack of international standardization), irritant reactions were not uncommon in practice. This was due to: (a) the nature of substances and/or mixtures applied to the skin, (b) a too-high concentration of some allergens, above the threshold of irritation.

Such irritant reactions may still occur nowadays, when inappropriate methodology is used (Fig. 3.9).

The clinical signs of irritant patch test reactions are varied, in relation with the nature and/or concentration of irritants [34].

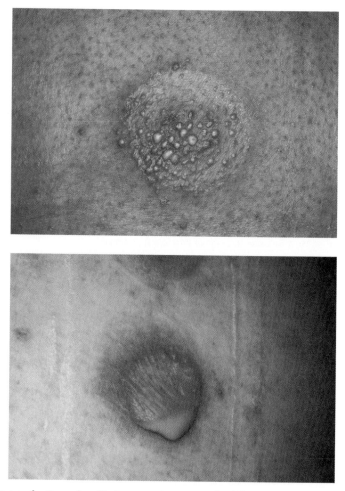

a

b

Fig. 3.9a, b. Examples of irritant reactions. **a** pustular follicular. **b** pustular diffuse

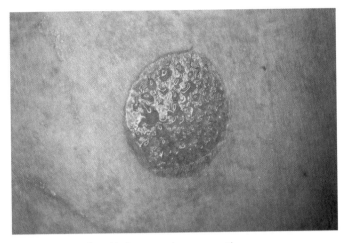

Fig. 3.9c. Examples of irritant reactions. **c** necrotic

They are classically described as follows:

a. Erythematous reactions

Erythema is strictly limited to the site of application of substances, with sharp, well delineated margins. This means that when a square patch test unit is used, erythema has a square shape. The reaction is sometimes discretely scaly, but usually not oedematous.

Allergens from the standard and/or additional series may provoke in some patients mild erythematous irritant reactions; they occur "at random" and are probably related to skin hypersensitivity in these patients.

Among allergens of the standard series, fragrance mix and thiuram mix are usually quoted as candidates for such marginal irritant reactions. In those cases, strategies to be applied for further patch testing are explained elsewhere (see Chap. 9).

b. Purpuric reactions

Purpuric patch test reactions are not uncommon with some allergens, in particular cobalt chloride. About 5% of patients tested with 1% cobalt chloride in petrolatum show this petechial haemorrhage. Histopathologic examination reveals slight perivascular lymphocytic infiltration, swollen endothelium, and extravasation of erythrocytes, mainly localized to the acrosyringium. Purpuric reactions can also be observed when patch testing with paraphenylenediamine, IPPD and some drugs.

c. "Soap or shampoo effect" reactions.

These are so named because they are typically produced by patch tests with soaps and detergents. The skin is red or slightly shiny and wrinkled; there are usually no vesicles; pruritus is uncommon. It is therefore never recommended to test with soaps or detergents. Such reactions may still occur with soluble oils (which do contain detergents), when the test concentration is inappropriate.

d. Blistering (or bullous) reactions

Blistering occurs after testing with non-diluted or overly concentrated caustic products, such as gasoline, kerosene and turpentine. Patch tests with quaternary ammonium salts may blister even when low concentrations are used.

e. Pustular reactions

These are sometimes consecutive to bullous reactions. Pustules are the result of an afflux of polymorphonuclear neutrophils (sterile pustules) or are less often due to superinfection (by staphylococci). In those circumstances, a unique large pustule is observed at the site of application.

Another type of pustular reaction may occur. The application area, uniformly erythematous, is dotted with small follicular pustules. This type of reaction mainly occurs with metallic salts (such as chromate, cobalt, nickel, copper) in atopic patients. The reaction can be exclusively irritant in nature, or be superimposed onto a true allergic reaction. Formerly, a similar pattern of reaction (purely irritant, non-allergic) was observed when croton oil was applied to the skin ("croton oil effect").

f. Necrotic or escharotic reactions

These are the most violent irritant reactions. For example, caustic soda or kerosene provoke such reactions.

3.10
False-Positive Patch Test Reactions

False-positive reactions can be defined as positive patch test reactions occurring in the absence of contact allergy [35–37]. These are manifold; nevertheless, the following list (Table 3.2) is mainly related to technical errors (which can be avoided) or to a misinterpretation of the test results, in particular when using inadequate concentrations of allergens.

Some of them are self-evident and can be predicted and monitored by the dermatologist carrying out patch testing, while others cannot.

3.11
False-Negative Patch Test Reactions

False-negative reactions can be defined as negative patch test reactions occurring in the presence of contact allergy [38]. The most common causes have been summarized in Table 3.3.

Table 3.2. False-positive patch test reactions

1	Too high a test concentration for a defined allergen
2	Impure or contaminated test substance
3	The vehicle is an irritant (especially solvents and very rarely petrolatum)
4	Excess of test preparation applied
5	The test substance, usually as crystals, is unevenly dispersed in the vehicle. This can occur when prepared at the hospital (i.e. not by manufacturers).
6	Current or recent dermatitis at test site
7	Current dermatitis at distant skin sites
8	Pressure effects of tapes, mechanical irritation of solid test materials, furniture and garments (see Sect. 3.14)
9	Adhesive tape reactions
10	The patch itself has caused reactions

Table 3.3. False-negative patch test reactions

1	Insufficient penetration of the allergen
	a) Too low a test concentration for a defined allergen
	b) The test substance is not released from the vehicle or retained by the filter paper
	c) Insufficient amount of test preparation applied
	d) Insufficient occlusion
	e) Duration of contact too brief; the test strip has fallen off or slipped
	f) The test was not applied to the recommended site the upper back
2	The reading is made too early; e.g. neomycin and corticosteroids are known to give delayed reactions
3	The test site has been treated with corticosteroids or irradiated with UV
4	Systemic treatment with corticosteroids or immunomodulators
5	Allergen is not in active form, insufficiently oxidized (oil of turpentine, rosin compounds, *d*-limonene) or degraded

Some of them are self-evident and can be predicted and monitored by the dermatologist, while others cannot. Examples of the latter category may arise when: (a) testing has been carried out in a refractory or "anergic" phase [39]; (b) the test does not reproduce the clinical exposure (multiple applications), where some adjuvant factors are present (sweating, friction, pressure, damaged skin), or penetration at the site is lower than that of clinical exposure (eyelids, axillae). A stripped skin technique is recommended in the latter case, where the test sites are stripped with tape before application of test preparations.

The differential diagnoses photoallergy and contact urticaria should also be considered.

3.12
Compound Allergy

The concept of "compound allergy", very popular among dermatologists, cannot *strictu sensu* be considered a false-positive or negative patch test reaction. It is the reason why it is described in a separate section.

The term "compound allergy" is used to describe the condition in patients who are patch test-positive to formulated products, usually cosmetic creams or topical medicaments, but test negative to all the ingredients tested individually [40]. This phenomenon can sometimes be explained by irritancy of the original formulation, but in some cases it has been demonstrated that the reactivity was due to the combination of the ingredients to form reaction products. Another reason might be that the ingredients were patch tested at the usage concentrations, which are too low for many allergens (e.g. MCI/MI, neomycin). Pseudo-compound allergy, due to faulty patch testing technique, is likely to be more common than true compound allergy. In a recent review [41], several proven or possible compound allergens were listed. The formation of allergenic reaction products can take place within the product ("chemical allergenic reactions") but also metabolically in the skin ("biological allergenic reactions") [41].

The "quenching phenomenon" is a consistent finding whereby cinnamic aldehyde alone induces sensitization, but when mixed with other fragrance compounds such as eugenol or *d*-limonene induces no sensitization. Patients who are sensitive to cinnamic aldehyde can sometimes tolerate perfumes containing this allergen because of presumed chemical changes (quenching) that occur during the usual aging process of a "mature" perfume.

3.13
Cross-Sensitization

In cross-sensitization, contact allergy caused by a primary allergen is combined with allergy to other chemically closely related substances. In those patients who have become sensitized to one substance, an allergic contact dermatitis can be provoked or worsened by several other related substances. A patient positive to *p*-phenylenediamine not only reacts to the dye itself, but also to immunochemically related substances which have an amino group in the para position, e.g. azo compounds, local anaesthetics and sulphonamides.

Cross-sensitization occurs among the methacrylates but not uniformly. Methyl methacrylate cannot be used as the sole screening monomer for acrylate sensitivity.

When studying cross-sensitization, it is essential to use pure test compounds.

3.14
Unwanted Adverse Reactions of Patch Testing

The greatest hazard is omission of patch testing procedures in the management of patients who have certain dermatoses. Such omission dooms these patients to repeated attacks of avoidable contact dermatitis [42].

Side effects of patch testing patients are listed in Table 3.4. Some of them are described in detail. Such unwanted effects are seldom encountered in daily practice. In this respect, it must be emphasized that the risk-benefit equation of patch testing is much in favour of the benefit.

Table 3.4. Unwanted adverse reactions of patch testing

Patch test sensitization	("Active sensitization") see Sect. 3.14.1
The excited skin syndrome	("Angry back") see Sect. 3.14.2
"Ectopic" flare of dermatitis	On rare occasions, a positive patch test reaction may be accompanied by a specific flare of an existing or pre-existing dermatitis that was caused by the test allergen. This side effect can be minimized by testing patients free of any current active dermatitis.
Persistence of a positive patch test reaction	A notorious patch test reaction for persisting for more than one month is that due to a 0.5% aqueous solution of gold chloride in a gold-sensitive patient. Its meaning is unknown.
Pressure effect	This consists of a red, usually depressed mark "imprinted" into the skin. It is a transient effect due to the application of solid materials. In practice, it can be due to: (a) the pressure of chamber's rings or squares. This is a physically-induced edge effect, distinct from the chemically-induced edge effect (see Sect. 3.8); (b) the use of allergens in a solid form (see Sect. 7.6.3).

Table 3.4 (continued)

The Koebner phenomenon	A positive patch test reaction in a patient who has active psoriasis or lichen planus may reproduce these dermatoses at the patch test site, during the weeks following patch test application [49]. The use of a topical corticosteroid usually quickly clears the lesion.
Hyperpigmentation	Hyperpigmentation from patch tests occurs infrequently and is most likely in darkly pigmented persons. If fades progressively after applying repeatedly topical cortico-steroids. Sunlight or artificial UV exposure, immediately following removal of patch tests especially to fragrance materials, leads to hyperpigmentation of patch test sites in relation with photosensitivity, as in berloque dermatitis. This side effect is more common in Oriental populations (see Sect. 3.15.2).
Hypopigmentation	Post-inflammatory hypopigmentation may occur at the sites of positive patch test reactions. It is usually a transient event (e.g. phenol).
Bacterial and viral infections	These adverse reactions have been occasionally described, but are exceedingly rare.
Necrosis, scarring and keloids	Foolhardy testing, with strong irritants (acids, alkalis, or chemicals of unknown composition) may produce such adverse reactions. Good practice of patch testing has entirely suppressed the occurrence of these complications, that are only of historical interest.
Anaphylactoid reactions	Anaphylactoid reactions or shock from, e.g. neomycin, bacitracin have been reported. These can be considered exceptional.

3.14.1
Patch Test Sensitization ("Active Sensitization")

By definition, a negative patch test reaction followed by a flare-up after 10–20 days, and then a positive reaction after 3 days at retesting, means that sensitization was induced by the patch procedure. There is a risk of active sensitization from the standard and/or additional series. Common examples are *p*-phenylenediamine, thiuram mix, epoxy resin, sesquiterpene lactone mix, primula extracts and, in recent years, isothiazolinone [43] or acrylates [44]. The risk, however, is uncommon when the testing is carried out according to internationally accepted guidelines. Sensitization by a patch test very rarely causes the patient any subsequent dermatitis or affects the course of a previous dermatitis.

It must be emphasized that the overall risk-benefit equation of patch testing patients is much in favour of the benefit. On the other hand, we advise against "prophetic" patch testing of non-dermatitic potential employees, because in that case the risk-benefit equation is very much in favour of the risk of active sensitization.

3.14.2
Excited Skin Syndrome ("Angry Back")

This represents a very important issue. Mitchell [45] used the term "angry back" to describe a regional phenomenon caused by the presence of a strongly positive reaction, a state of skin hyperreactivity in which other patch test sites become reactive, especially to marginal irritants, such as formaldehyde and potassium dichromate. He believed that these concomitant "positive" reactions cannot be relied on. Indeed, when retesting, these reactions were negative. He suggested that the true index of sensitivity was falsely exaggerated by concomitant patch testing. Nickel sulphate and potassium dichromate were considered best examples of such false-positive reactions. To confirm or deny the significance of individual reactions found on the "angry back," he recommended sequential testing later with each substance alone.

Because patch test may be performed elsewhere besides the back, Maibach and Mitchell [46, 47] broadened the term "angry back" to the "excited skin syndrome" (ESS), which was extensively reviewed later on [48]. The pathogenesis of ESS has not yet been clearly elucidated.

When in doubt about the occurrence of ESS in a patient, the strategy to be conducted is individual *sequential retesting,* with each incriminated allergen, preferably on a different skin site. This procedure can be completed by additional tests, such as ROAT tests (see 7.4). It is a matter of the utmost importance in medico-legal situations.

It is our experience that the ESS is less frequent nowadays, possibly for two main reasons: (a) patch testing only on intact skin in patients free of any current dermatitis; (b) using smaller amounts of allergens, in relation with new patch test units (chambers).

The ESS is distinct from the "status eczematicus," contrary to what is written in most textbooks on contact dermatitis. Status eczematicus means that, at many patch test sites, there are positive non-specific reactions, due to a state of skin hypersensitivity. This does occur when general rules of patch testing are not respected, such as patch testing patients with active atopic dermatitis or other types of dermatitis. Status eczematicus makes reading impossible; it can be avoided by using correct procedures.

3.15
Patch Test Readings in Different Ethnic Populations

Most publications dealing with patch test readings refer to Caucasian populations. It seems important to know whether differences may occur when reading patch test results in different ethnic populations.

3.15.1
Patch Test Reading in Oriental Populations

Particular Aspects of Reading

The skin colour in Oriental races (Japanese, Chinese, Korean, etc.) varies from white fair skin (equivalent to Fitzpatrick classification type II to IV) to dark complexion (equivalent to Fitzpatrick classification skin types V and VI).

For dark-skinned individuals (skin types V and VI), skin marking of patch test sites is important because by the 2nd and 4th day, it is often difficult to identify the location of the patch test sites. Special markers incorporating silver nitrate (though it may cause irritant reactions) may be more effective than marking the skin test sites in a conventional way. Goh in Singapore uses the following marker solution:

- Gentian violet 1%
- Meth Spirit (95%) 50%
- Silver nitrate 20%
- Distilled water to 100%

The fluorescence skin marker is an alternative.

For fair skin (type II to type IV), a patch test reaction is not difficult to interpret. Allergic patch test reactions are usually easily discernible. The erythema, papules and mild oedema of allergic patch test reactions is usually very obvious in skin types II and III. In darker skin types (types V and VI), a mild positive allergic patch test reaction may be overlooked as the erythema may not be obvious. However, the oedema and papules/vesicles are usually obvious and palpable.

In darker skin of Malays and Indians, allergic patch test reactions may be difficult to discern. Erythema is barely visible. Much will have to depend on the appearance of papules/vesicles and oedema. Palpation of the patch test site may help to detect allergic reactions. Associated pruritus on papular eruptions on the patch test site helps to affirm the possibility of the presence of a positive allergic patch test reaction.

Pigmented Contact Dermatitis

Pigmented contact dermatitis is a particular entity characterized by a diffuse brown, slate-coloured, greyish-brown, reddish-brown, or bluish-brown pigmentation. It occurs in the weeks following an acute episode of irritant or allergic contact dermatitis [50]. Pigmented contact dermatitis is rare in Caucasians but not uncommon in Mongoloids. Most recent cases have been reported from Japan. Various allergens have been incriminated, namely Naphthol AS, 1 phenyl-azo-2 naphthol, trichlorocarban, parabens, jasmine oil, rose oil, benzylsalicylate and musk ambrette [51, 52]. Positive patch tests to these allergens become hyperpigmented in the days or weeks following patch test application [51, 52] and remain so for long periods of time.

3.15.2
Patch Test Reading in Black Populations

It is surprising that in most textbooks of contact dermatitis, no mention is made about particular aspects of patch test reading in black populations. In practice, reading does not cause insurmountable difficulties.

Two specific points deserve special attention:

1. Erythema is distinctly visible in some cases, or may present itself as a darker black hue in some others.
2. In black skin, vesicles of eczematous reactions (including positive patch test reactions) do not tend to burst readily; since they exhibit a yellowish hue, they can be confounded with tiny pustules (Fig. 3.10). This particular aspect is certainly related to the fact that, in black skin, the stratum corneum has more cell layers and requires more tape strips to remove it compared to Caucasoid stratum corneum [53].

The darker the skin, the more difficult it is to mark. For very dark skin, a fluorescent marking ink is probably best, the dots being located by a Wood's light in a dark room [54].

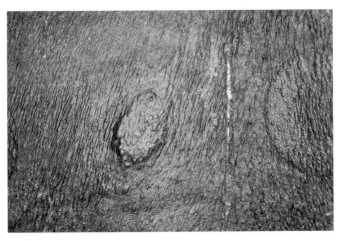

Fig. 3.10. Positive allergic patch test reaction on black skin. Vesicles exhibit a yellowish hue

3.16
Patch Testing Techniques in Different Climatic Environments

The patch testing procedures should be modified in different climatic conditions. This is because of the adherence of the tape and moisture of the skin surface under different climatic environments.

3.16.1
Temperate Climates

In some temperate countries, patch testing is carried out only during the cooler seasons and discontinued during summer time, because the hot humid climate in summer may cause the tape to be dislodged more readily and patients generally find it uncomfortable to have strips of tape left on their skin for 48 h.

In many places, there is no real need to interrupt patch testing activities during summer time. The only reason why this habit does occur is for practical convenience, in relation with personnel holidays.

Useful information is related to seasonal variations in patch test reading in temperate countries [55].

- Chapping of the skin during winter predisposes to irritant contact dermatitis and also increases the incidence of false-positive reactions to substances such as formaldehyde, mercurials and propyleneglycol.
- Some authors found many positive reactions in summer, but far fewer during cooler weather. Thus, occlusion and sweating may increase the number of positive reactions to some substances, whereas propyleneglycol, which is hygroscopic, and some other marginal irritants may often appear to be more of an irritant in winter [55].

3.16.2
Tropical Climates

Allergic contact dermatitis from whatever cause can be aggravated by environmental factors such as heat, high humidity and dust [55].

In the tropics where there is little seasonable variation, there is no "ideal" season when patch testing can be done most comfortably. Patch testing is usually carried out throughout the year. Because of the high ambient temperature and high humidity, the patch testing procedure may need some modification to ensure that the occlusive effects of the patch test chamber are maintained and that patients comply with the instructions carefully.

In addition, because of the higher ambient temperature it is recommended that the patch test allergens be stored in a cool place when not in use. The test allergens should be kept in a refrigerator.

3.16.3
Patch Testing Procedures in the Tropics

The warm humid environment in the tropics makes patch testing an uncomfortable experience for the patients. Miliaria can occur at the sites of patch testing, due to occlusion. Patients should be given clear instructions on the patch testing procedures.

Instructions for Patient

To ensure compliance, the following instructions may be given to the patients:

- Patients will be allowed to continue to take light showers to clean their face, chest, limbs, lower torso. They should avoid washing the back (patch test sites) with water.
- The back where the patch test tapes are placed will be allowed to be cleaned daily with light moist towels, avoiding the test strips area.
- Patients should avoid outdoor activities and remain in a cool air-conditioned environment whenever possible.

Technical Adaptations

Patch testing can be carried out with the various patch test chambers available commercially. The Finn chambers are widely used for patch testing in the tropics. However, the hot, humid environment causes sweating and makes plaster adhesion to the skin poor. Patch test plasters tend to come off easily. Reinforcement of the patch test plaster is useful to ensure proper occlusion. An effective way is to reinforce strips of plasters on the edges of the patch test tapes.

The conventional skin marker does not remain on the skin due to perspiration. The silver nitrate skin marker is a useful marker for identifying patch test sites.

References

1. Adams RM (1993) Profiles of greats in contact dermatitis. I Jozef Jadassohn (1863–1936). Am J Contact Dermatitis 4:58–59
2. Jadassohn J (1896) Zur Kenntnis der medikamentösen Dermatosen. Verhandlungen der Deutschen Dermatologischen Gesellschaft, Fünfter Congress, Graz, 1895. Wilhelm Braunmüller, Wien, Leipzig, pp 103–129
3. Gallant CJ (1994) Patch testing a century later. In: Hogan DJ (ed) Occupational skin disorders. Ikagu-Shoin, New York Tokyo, pp 41–53
4. Rietschel RL, Fowler JF Jr (2001) Fisher's contact dermatitis, 5th edn. Lippincott Williams and Wilkins, Philadelphia, p 9
5. Grob JJ, Sambuc R, Gouvernet J (1997) Introduction to epidemiology and prevention in dermatology. In: Grob JJ, Stern RS, MacKie RM, Weinstock WA (eds) Epidemiology, causes and prevention of skin diseases. Blackwell Science, Oxford, p 6
6. Pirilä V (1975) Chamber test versus patch test for epicutaneous testing. Contact Dermatitis 1:48–52
7. Lachapelle JM, Douka MA (1985) An evaluation of the compatibility between aluminium Finn Chambers and various mercurials dissolved in water or dispersed in petrolatum. Dermatosen 33:12–14
8. Böhler-Sommeregger K, Lindemayr H (1986) Contact sensitivity to aluminium. Contact Dermatitis 15:278–281
9. Dooms-Goossens A (1982) Allergic contact dermatitis to ingredients used in topical applied pharmaceutical products and cosmetics. Katholieke Universiteit, Leuven, Belgium, Thesis
10. de Groot AC (1994) Patch testing. Test concentrations and vehicles for 3700 chemicals, 2nd edn. Elsevier, Amsterdam
11. Patch Test Products Catalogue (2001) Chemotechnique Diagnostics
12. Benezra C, Andanson J, Chabeau G, Ducombs G, Foussereau J, Lachapelle JM, Lacroix M, Martin P (1978) Concentrations of patch test allergens: are we comparing the same things? Contact Dermatitis 4:103–105
13. Sukanto H, Nater JP, Bleumink E (1981) Influence of topically applied corticosteroids on patch test reactions. Contact Dermatitis 7:180–185

14. O'Quinn SE, Isbell RH (1969) Effect of oral prednisone on eczema patch test reactions, Arch Dermatol 99:380–389

15. Sjövall P (1988) Ultraviolet radiation and allergic contact dermatitis. An experimental and clinical study. Thesis, University of Lund, Sweden

16. Lindelöf B, Lidén S, Lagerholm B (1985) The effect of grenz rays on the expression of allergic contact dermatitis in man. Scand J Immunol 21:463–469

17. Goossens A, Neyens K, Vigan M (2001) Contact allergy in children. In: Rycroft RJG, Menné T, Frosch PJ, Lepoittevin JP (eds) Textbook of contact dermatitis, 3rd edn. Springer, Berlin Heidelberg New York, pp 581–603

18. Vigan M (2002) Contact allergy in children. Contact Dermatitis 46 [Suppl 4]: S13–S14

19. Fischer T, Maibach HI (1986) Patch testing in allergic contact dermatitis: an update. Semin Dermatol 5:214–224

20. Wahlberg JE, Wahlberg ENG (1987) Quantification of skin blood flow at patch test sites. Contact Dermatitis 17:229–233

21. Uter WJC, Geier J, Schnuch A (1996) Good clinical practice in patch testing: readings beyond day 2 are necessary: a confirmatory analysis. Am J Contact Dermatitis 7:231–237

22. Saino M, Rinara P, Guarrera M (1995) Reading patch tests on day 7. Contact Dermatitis 32:312

23. Todd DJ, Handley J, Metwali M, Allen GE, Burrows D (1996) Day 4 is better than day 3 for a single patch test reading. Contact Dermatitis 34:402–404

24. Geier J, Gefeller O, Wiechmann K, Fuchs T (1999) Patch test reactions at D4, D5 and D6. Contact Dermatitis 40:119–126

25. Manuskiatti W, Maibach HI (1996) 1 versus 2 and 3-day diagnostic patch testing. Contact Dermatitis 35:197–200

26. Goh CL, Wong WK, Ng SK (1994) Comparison between 1-day and 2-day occlusion times in patch testing. Contact Dermatitis 31:48–49

27. le Coz CJ, Muller B (2002) A practical sparkling and durable way to mark patch test sites. Contact Dermatitis 46 [Suppl 4]:552–553

28. Wilkinson DS, Fregert S, Magnusson B, Bandmann HJ, Calnan CD, Cronin E, Hjorth N, Maibach HI, Malten KE, Meneghini CL, Pirilä V (1970) Terminology of contact dermatitis. Acta Dermato-Venereologica 50:287

29. Lachapelle JM (2001) Histopathological and immunohistopathological features of allergic and irritant contact dermatitis. In: Rycroft RJG, Menné T, Frosch RJ, Lepoittevin JP (eds) Textbook of contact dermatitis, 3rd edn. Springer, Berlin Heidelberg New York, pp 159–171

30. Lachapelle JM, Tennstedt D, Fyad A, Masmoudi ML, Nouaigui H (1988) Ring-shaped positive patch test reactions to allergens in liquid vehicles. Contact Dermatitis 18:234–236

31. Fyad A, Masmoudi ML, Lachapelle JM (1987) The "edge effect" with patch test materials. Contact Dermatitis 16:147–151

32. Isaksson M, Brandao FM, Bruze M, Goossens A (2000) Recommendations to include budesonide and tixocortol pivalate in the European standard series. Contact Dermatitis 43:41–42

33. Lachapelle JM (1989) A left versus right side comparison study of Epiquick® patch test reactions in 100 consecutive patients. Contact Dermatitis 20: 51–56

34. Foussereau J, Benezra C, Maibach HI (1982) Occupational contact dermatitis. Clinical and chemical aspects. Munksgaard, Copenhagen, pp 26–27

35. Fregert S (1981) Manual of contact dermatitis. Munksgaard, Copenhagen, pp 77–78

36. Rycroft RJG (1986) False reactions to nonstandard patch tests. Semin Dermatol 5:225–230

37. Wahlberg JE (2001) Patch testing. In: Rycroft RJG, Menné T, Frosch PJ, Lepoittevin JP (eds) Textbook of contact dermatitis, 3rd edn. Springer, Berlin Heidelberg New York, p 454

38. Wahlberg JE (2001) Patch testing. In: Rycroft RJG, Menné T, Frosch PJ, Lepoittevin JP (eds) Textbook of contact dermatitis, 3rd edn. Springer, Berlin Heidelberg New York, p 456

39. Bruynzeel DP, Maibach HI (1990) Excited skin syndrome and the hyporeactive state: current status. In Menné T, Maibach HI (eds) Exogenous dermatoses: environmental dermatitis. CRC Press, Boca Raton, pp 141–150

40. Kelett JK, Ring CH, Beck MH (1986) Compound allergy to medicaments. Contact Dermatitis 14:45–48

41. Bashir SJ, Maibach HI (1997) Compound allergy. An overview. Contact Dermatitis 36:179–183

42. Rietschel RL, Fowler JF Jr (2001) Fisher's contact dermatitis, 5th edn. Lippincott Williams and Wilkins, Philadelphia, pp 13–18

43. Björkner B, Bruze M, Dahlquist I, Fregert S, Gruvberger B, Persson K (1986) Contact allergy to the preservative Kathon® CG. Contact Dermatitis 14: 85–90

44. Kanerva L, Estlander T, Jolanki R (1988) Sensitization to patch test acrylates. Contact Dermatitis 18:10–15

45. Mitchell JC (1975) The angry back syndrome. Eczema creates eczema. Contact Dermatitis 1:193–194

46. Maibach HI (1981) The ESS-excited skin syndrome (alias the "angry back") In: Ring J, Burg G (eds) New trends in allergy. Springer, Berlin Heidelberg New York, pp 208–221

47. Mitchell JC, Maibach HI (1982) The angry back syndrome: the excited skin syndrome. Semin Dermatol 1:9

48. Bruynzeel DP, Maibach HI (1986) Excited skin syndrome (angry back). Arch Dermatol 122:323–328

49. Weiss G, Shemer A, Trau H (2002) The Koebner phenomenon: review of the literature JEADV 16:241–248

50. Nakayama H (2001) Pigmented contact dermatitis and chemical depigmentation. In: Rycroft RJG, Menné T, Frosch PJ, Lepoittevin JP (eds) Textbook of contact dermatitis, 3rd edn. Springer, Berlin Heidelberg New York, pp 381–401

51. Hayakawa R, Matsunaga K, Kojima S et al (1985) Naphthol AS as a cause of pigmented contact dermatitis. Contact Dermatitis 13:20–25

52. Hayakawa R, Matsunaga K, Arima Y (1987) Airborne pigmented contact dermatitis due to musk ambrette in incense. Contact Dermatitis 16:96–98

53. Weigand DA, Haygood C, Gaylor JR (1974) Cell layers and density of Negro and Caucasian stratum corneum. J Invest Dermatol 62:563–568

54. Cronin E (1980) Contact dermatitis. Churchill Livingstone, Edinburgh, p 5

55. Wilkinson JD, Shaw S (1998) Contact dermatitis: allergic. In: Champion RH et al (eds) Rook, Wilkinson, Ebling, Textbook of dermatology, 6th edn. Blackwell Science, Oxford, p 746

56. Okoro A, Rook AJ, Canizares O (1992) Eczemas in the tropics. Plant dermatitis. In: Canizares O, Harman R (eds) Clinical tropical dermatology, 2nd edn. Blackwell Science, Oxford, pp 449–481

CHAPTER 4

The Standard and Additional Series of Patch Tests

J.-M. LACHAPELLE

4.1
Historical Background

The use of a standard series in all tested patients was adopted worldwide in the 1980s. Formerly, many authors refused to adhere to its systematic use and championed the concept of "selected patch tests". Werner Jadassohn (at Geneva) had a strong influence on many colleagues in this respect. The principle of "choice" or "selection" was based upon a careful recording of anamnestic data, especially in the field of occupational dermatology [1]. A similar view was shared in France by Foussereau [2]. Their opinion was that "testing systematically" with a standard series led unavoidably to a lazy clinical attitude. They argued that by doing so, clinicians were tempted to neglect the medical history of each individual patient.

Conversely, the standard series found enthusiastic defenders among renowned pioneers in the field of allergic contact dermatitis.

Bruno Bloch acted as a group leader for promoting and disseminating the idea of applying a limited standard series on each patient [3]. This was made in close connection with Jozef Jadassohn in Breslau (Bloch's former teacher when he was in Bern), Blumenthal and Jaffé in Berlin, and later Sulzberger in New York.

Poul Bonnevie, Professor of Occupational Medicine in Copenhagen, expanded Bloch's embryonic standard series of tests and published it in his famous textbook of environmental dermatology [4]. The list (21 allergens) can be considered the prototype of the standard series of patch tests. Later, this list of allergens was modified and updated by the founding members of the ICDRG group. The changes were based on the experience of the members in their own countries and mirrored the findings and current situation in different parts of Europe and the United States.

<hr>

4.2
Advantages and Disadvantages of Using a Standard Series of Patch Tests

4.2.1
Advantages

- The standard series corresponds to an allergological check-up of each individual patient, as regards the most common allergens encountered in the environment. Positive and negative patch test results map out the allergological profile of the patient.
- The standard series compensates for anamnestic failures. Even when the clinician tries to record carefully the history of each individual patient, he may omit important events in some cases, despite using a detailed standardized questionnaire. Positive patch test results lead the clinician to ask some additional (retrospective) questions.
- The systematic use of the standard series permits comparative studies in different countries, thus increasing our knowledge in terms of geographic variations.

<hr>

4.2.2
Disadvantages

- The standard series can produce a "sleeping" effect on the clinician's attitude. This perverse result is avoided when the standard series is considered a limited technical tool, representing one of the pieces of a puzzle, to be combined with other means of diagnosis. The general principle to be kept in mind is that the standard series cannot replace a detailed anamnestic (and catamnestic) investigation.
- Theoretically, the application of the standard series could induce an active sensitization to some allergens. Common examples are *p*-phenylenediamine, primin, and isothiazolinone [5]. The risk, however, is extremely low when testing is carried out according to internationally accepted guidelines.

In conclusion, taking into account all these considerations, it must be emphasized that the overall risk–benefit equation of patch testing patients with the allergens of the standard series is much in favour of the benefit [5].

4.3
The Three Major Standard Series Used Throughout the World

There is no unanimity worldwide as regards the contents of a standard series. There are three major options in building a standard series, in relation with regional potential variations:

1. The revised European standard series, as recommended by the European Environmental and Contact Dermatitis Research Group (EEC-DRG) [6], in 2001 (22 allergens + primin, optional)
2. The North American standard series according to the North American Contact Dermatitis Group (20 allergens)
3. The Japanese standard series according to the Japanese Society for Contact Dermatitis (25 allergens)

A comparison of the three lists (Table 4.1) suggests that 33 allergens are potentially considered in the international standardization process. Note that neomycin sulphate in lists (a) and (b) of Table 4.1 is synonymous with fradiomycin sulphate in list (c).

The discrepancies in comparing lists (a), (b), and (c) are due to two main factors:

1. There are regional variations, related to either the natural occurrence of allergens (e.g. urushiol) or to a significant variability in the use of some allergens in various regions, due to different medical, cosmetic, industrial, or environmental habits.
2. A different approach of the three research groups (or societies) regarding each individual allergen, thus reaching dissimilar conclusions. The three groups are working independently, and have not shared their opinions so as to reach a worldwide consensus.

Most decisions reached by each group are partly based upon multicentre studies and/or thorough literature reviews.

Table 4.1. Comparative lists of allergens in three different standard series

Compound	EECDRG[a] %	NACDG[b] %	JCDS[c] %
1. Potassium dichromate	0.5	0.25	0.5
2. Neomycin sulphate	20	20	–
3. Thiuram mix	1	1	1.25
4. *p*-Phenylenediamine base	1	1	1
5. Cobalt chloride ($CoCl_2$ $6H_2O$)	1	–	1
6. Benzocaine	5	5	–
7. Formaldehyde	1 (aq.)	1 (aq.)	1 (aq.)
8. Colophony	20	20	20 (rosin)
9. Clioquinol	5	–	–
10. Balsam of Peru (Myroxylon Pereirae)	25	25	25
11. *N*-Isopropyl-*N*-phenyl paraphenylenediamine (IPPD)	0.1	–	–
12. Wool (lanolin) alcohols	30	30	30
13. Mercapto mix	2	1	2
14. Epoxy resin	1	1	1
15. Paraben mix	16	–	15
16. *p-tert*-Butylphenol formaldehyde (BPF) resin	1	1	1
17. Fragrance mix	8	–	8
18. Quaternium 15	1	2	–
19. Nickel sulphate ($NiSO_4$ $6H_2O$)	5	2.5	2.5
20. Cl+Me-isothiazolinone	0.01 (aq.)	–	0.01 (aq.)
21. Mercaptobenzothiazole (MBT)	2	1	–
22. Sesquiterpene lactone mix	0.1	–	–
23. Primin	0.01	–	0.01
24. Imidazolidinyl urea	–	2 (aq.)	–
25. Cinnamic aldehyde	–	1	–
26. Carba mix	–	3	–

Table 4.1 (continued)

Compound	EECDRG[a] %	NACDG[b] %	JCDS[c] %
27. Ethylenediamine dihydrochloride	–	1	1
28. Black rubber (PPD)	–	0.6	0.6
29. Fradiomycin sulphate	–	–	20
30. Caine mix	–	–	7
31. Dithiocarbamate mix	–	–	2
32. Urushiol	–	–	0.002
33. Thimerosal (thiomersal)	–	–	0.1
34. Ammoniated mercuric chloride	–	–	1
35 Petrolatum	–	–	As is

[a] The revised European standard series as recommended by the European Environmental and Contact Dermatitis Research Group, 2001. The concentrations quoted refer to petrolatum unless otherwise stated.
[b] North American standard series according to the North American Contact Dermatitis Research Group. The concentrations quoted refer to petrolatum unless otherwise stated.
[c] The Japanese standard series according to the Japanese Society for Contact Dermatitis. The concentrations quoted refer to petrolatum unless otherwise stated.

4.4
Some Remarks About the "Mixes" of the Standard Series

The basic idea of using mixes instead of single allergens is to save time and space. In this respect, patients are tested with a number of closely related substances. The screening capacity of the standard series is thereby greatly increased. Nevertheless, the value of these mixes is sometimes questioned. It is difficult to find an optimal concentration for each allergen in a common vehicle (usually petrolatum) and to determine whether the allergens metabolize or interact to potentiate or quench a reaction [7].

It is recommended that patients positive for a mix be retested with the individual ingredients. Infrequently, the latter results are negative, and in that case it is questioned whether the initial reaction was an expression of irritancy and/or the ingredients have interacted. The opposite has also been noticed. The patient may be negative to a particular mix, but reacts when retested with its ingredients.

The composition of the various mixes of the standard series is detailed in Table 4.2 [6].

Table 4.2. The composition of the mixes of the European Standard Series

Thiuram mix	1% pet.
Dipentamethylenethiuram disulphide (0.25%)	
Tetramethylthiuram disulphide (0.25%)	
Tetraethylthiuram disulphide (0.25%)	
Tetramethylthiuram monosulphide (0.25%)	
Mercapto mix	2% pet.
N-Cyclohexylbenzothiazyl sulphenamide (0.5%)	
Dibenzothiazyl disulphide (0.5%)	
Mercaptobenzothiazole (0.5%)	
Morpholinyl mercaptobenzothiazole (0.5%)	
Fragrance mix (incl. 5% sorbitan sesquioleate)	8% pet.
α-Amylcinnamaldehyde(1%)	
Cinnamaldehyde (1%)	
Cinnamyl alcohol (1%)	
Eugenol (1%)	
Geraniol (1%)	
Hydroxycitronellal (1%)	
Isoeugenol (1%)	
Oak moss absolute (Evernia Prunastri) (1%)	
Paraben mix	16% pet.
Butylparaben (4%)	
Ethylparaben (4%)	
Methylparaben (4%)	
Propylparaben (4%)	
Sesquiterpene lactone mix	0.1% pet.
Alantolactone (0.033%)	
Dehydrocostus lactone (0.033%)	
Costunolide (0.033%)	

4.5
Proposal for an ICDRG Revised International Series of Patch Tests

Considering the current status of the standard series throughout the world, the members of the International Contact Dermatitis Research Group (ICDRG) discussed the possibility of using a shortened list of common allergens, that could be used internationally as a "minimal international standard series" [8].

Table 4.3 shows the allergens that have been considered eligible candidates for such a list.

4.6
List of Allergens Proposed for an Extended ICDRG Series
Which May Be Required According to Each Individual Situation

Some allergens present in one (or more) of the three lists of Table 4.1 are not considered eligible candidates for the revised international standard series presented in Table 4.3.

On the other hand, they are listed in an "extended series" (Table 4.4). Other allergens are also proposed in the extended series, since they are considered useful in the literature.

4.7
List of Allergens Proposed to Be Deleted from the Revised
and Extended ICDRG Series

Some of the allergens recorded in Table 4.1 lack general interest, for different reasons. Therefore, they are not proposed as candidates for an extended international series. Nevertheless, they could be used in specific circumstances.

These allergens, dispersed in petrolatum, are as follows: N-isopropyl-N-phenylparaphenylenediamine (IPPD) 0.1%; cinnamic aldehyde 1%; carba mix 3% (often lacks clinical relevance); black rubber (PPD) mix 0.6%; caïne mix 7%; dithiocarbamate mix 2%; ammoniated mercuric chloride 1%.

Table 4.3. Proposed allergens for a modified international standard series (concentrations refer to petrolatum unless otherwise stated)

	Concentration (%)
1. Potassium dichromate	0.5
2. Neomycin sulphate	20
3. Thiuram mix[a]	1
4. *p*-Phenylenediamine base (PPD)[b]	1
5. Formaldehyde	1 (aq.)
6. Colophony	20
7. Balsam of Peru	25
8. Wool (lanolin) alcohols	30
9. Mercapto mix[c]	1
10. Epoxy resin	1
11. *p-tert*-Butylphenol formaldehyde (BPF) resin	1
12. Fragrance mix[d]	8
13. Nickel sulphate ($NiSO_4 \cdot 6H_2O$)	2.5
14. Mercaptobenzothiazole (MBT)[e]	1
15. Budesonide[f]	0.1
16. Quaternium 15[g]	2
17. Cl+Me-isothiazolinone[h]	0.01 (aq.)
18. Imidazolidinyl urea	2 (aq.)
19. Tixocortol pivalate	1
20. Dibromodicyanobutane[i]	0.1

[a] Thiuram mix lacks high specificity and sensitivity.

[b] Some cases of hair dye dermatitis could be missed with the use of PPD alone.

[c] Mercapto mix lacks high specificity and sensitivity. The 1% mix, used in the North American standard series, is chosen since its stability has been proven by Hermal and approved by the FDA.

[d] If positive, breakdown is needed.

[e] MBT can identify cases of allergic contact dermatitis negative to mercapto mix, and vice versa.

[f] Despite its absence in the three standard series, budesonide is highly recommended in an international standard series, since it is considered an important marker for corticosteroid allergy [9].

[g] It is an important allergen in the United Kingdom, while it is not used in Japan.

[h] Mainly used in Japan.

[i] Synonym, dibromo-2,4-dicyanobutane 1,2-; methyldibromoglutaronitrile. Present in Euxyl K 400 (dibromodicyanobutane + phenoxyethanol 1:4)

Table 4.4. Proposed allergens for an extended international standard series (concentrations refer to petrolatum unless otherwise stated)

	Concentration (%)
A. Allergens present in one (or more) of the three lists of Table 4.1	
1. Cobalt chloride ($CoCl_2$ $6H_2O$)[a]	1
2. Benzocaine	5
3. Clioquinol	5
4. Paraben mix	16
5. Primin	0.01
6. Ethylenediamine dihydrochloride	1
7. Urushiol	0.002
8. Thimerosal (thiomersal)	0.1
B. Additional useful allergens	
9. Sesquiterpene lactone mix	0.1
10. Hydrocortisone 17-butyrate	1 (alc.)
11. 2,5 Diazolidinylurea[b]	2 (aq.)
12. Cetylstearylalcohol	20
13. Toluenesulphonamide formaldehyde resin	10
14. Propylene glycol	10 (aq.)

[a] Cobalt is not traced as relevant in many cases. Petechial reactions should not be read as positive.

[b] It is not used in Japan.

4.8
Succinct Information About Allergens

Some basic information about allergens proposed for an ICDRG revised international series of patch tests (see Sect. 4.5) as well as for an extended ICDRG series (see Sect. 4.6) is given here. More details are available in textbooks of contact dermatitis listed in the general references section at the end of this book. We have illustrated in Fig. 4.1 numerous positive patch test reactions in a multisensitized patient.

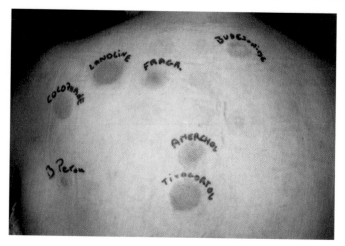

Fig. 4.1. Multisensitized patient. Multiple positive allergic patch test reactions

---

4.8.1
Allergens Listed in Sect. 4.5

1. Potassium dichromate
   Hexavalent form of chromium. Present in cement, tanning of leather, textile dyes, wood preservatives, alloys in metallurgy, safety matches, photography, electroplating, anticorrosives, ceramics, tattoos, paints, glues, pigments, detergents, and other materials.

2. Neomycin sulphate
   Broad-spectrum antibiotic in topical creams, powders, ointments, eye and ear drops. Growth promoter in veterinary use.

3. Thiuram mix
   Mixture of thiurams, used as rubber accelerators and vulcanizers, fungicides, disinfectants for seed, animal repellents, etc. (see Table 4.2).

4. *p*-Phenylenediamine (PPD)
   Primary intermediate in permanent hair dyes and fur dyes. Also used in photographic developers, lithography, photocopying, oils, greases, gasoline, and as antioxidant/accelerator in the rubber and plastic industries.

5. Formaldehyde
   Ubiquitous allergen. Used as astringent, disinfectant, preservative in cosmetics, metalworking fluids, shampoos, etc.
   Widespread use in several industrial procedures. Its presence in end-products can be checked by a specific spot test (see Sect. 7.8.2). There are many formaldehyde releasers.

6. Colophony
   Yellow resin in the production of varnishes, printing inks, paper, soldering fluxes, cutting fluids, glue tackifiers, adhesives, surface coatings, polish, waxes, cosmetics, topical medicaments, etc.

7. Balsam of Peru
   Flavour in tobacco, drinks, pastries, cakes, wines, liquors and spices. Fixative and fragrance in perfumery. In topical medicaments, dentistry, etc.

8. Wool alcohols
   Different types of alcohols (aliphatic, steroid, triterpenoid) present in wool fat (lanolin). As ointment base in cosmetic and pharmaceutical products.

9. Mercapto mix
   Mixture of mercaptothiazoles (see mercaptobenzothiazole and Table 4.2).

10. Epoxy resin
    Resin, based on epichlorhydrin and bisphenol A for use in adhesives, surface coatings, electrical insulation, plasticizers, polymer stabilizers, laminates, surface coatings, paints and inks, product finishers, PVC products and vinyl gloves. Oligomers may vary in molecular weight from 340 and higher. The higher the molecular weight, the less sensitizing the compound.

11. p-tert-Butylphenol formaldehyde (BPF) resin
    Resin used in adhesives for shoes and watch straps. Many other uses in various industrial procedures.

12. Fragrance mix
    Mixture of fragrances (see Table 4.2).

13. Nickel sulphate
    Nickel metal: a common allergen present in various alloys, electroplated metal, earrings, watches, buttons, zippers, rings, utensils, tools,

instruments, batteries, machinery parts, working solutions of metal cutting fluids, nickel plating for alloys, coins, pigments, orthopaedic plates, keys, scissors, razors, spectacle frames, kitchenware, etc.

14. Mercaptobenzothiazole

Accelerator, retarder and peptizer for natural and other rubber products. Fungicide. Corrosion inhibitor in soluble cutting oils and antifreeze mixtures. Also used in many other industrial procedures.

15. Budesonide

Non-halogenated corticosteroid for use in topical preparations and for the treatment of rhinitis and asthma. Belongs to the group B (triamcinolone acetonide) type of corticosteroids. One of the markers of corticosteroid allergy.

16. Quaternium 15

Formaldehyde-releaser used chiefly as a cosmetic preservative. Also in widespread usage in industry and household products. Marketed under different trade names.

17. Cl+Me-isothiazolinone

Used as a preservative in oils and cooling fluids, soaps, latex emulsions, slime control in paper mills, jet fluids, printing inks, detergents, shampoos, hair conditioners and bubble baths. Known also under the trade name Kathon CG. Many other trade names are indexed.

18. Imidazolidinyl urea

Formaldehyde-releaser used as a cosmetic preservative (lotions, creams, hair conditioners, shampoos, deodorants) and also in topical drugs. Known also under the trade name Germall 115 (not exclusive).

19. Tixocortol pivalate

Topical corticosteroid belonging to the group A (hydrocortisone) type of steroids used in nasal sprays for the treatment of rhinitis. Good marker for group A corticosteroid contact allergy.

20. Dibromodicyanobutane

Preservative for cosmetics, metalworking fluids, adhesives, latex emulsions and paints, dispersed pigments and detergents. Ingredient (with phenoxyethanol) in Euxyl K 400. Synonym: methyldibromoglutaronitrile.

4.8.2
Allergens Listed in Sect. 4.6

1. Cobalt chloride
   Component in paints for glass and porcelain. Siccative in paints. Present in various alloys.

2. Benzocaine
   Topical anaesthetic used in many over-the-counter preparations and/or topical drugs.

3. Cioquinol
   Synthetic anti-infective (antibacterial and to a lesser extent antifungal) agent. Present in topical drugs (i.e. Vioform). Occasionally used as a systemic drug.

4. Paraben mix
   Mixture of parabens (esters of parahydroxybenzoic acid) very widely used as preservatives in foods, drugs and cosmetics (see Table 4.2).

5. Primin
   Primin (or 2-methoxy-6 pentylbenzoquinone) is the major allergen in *Primula* dermatitis.

6. Ethylenediamine dihydrochloride
   Stabilizer in some steroid creams and rubber latex. Inhibitor in antifreeze solutions and cooling fluids. Component in aminophylline. One of the allergens in Mycolog cream.

7. Urushiol
   Oleoresin of the sap of the *Toxicodendron* plants. It contains catechols, which are the sensitizing chemicals.

8. Thimerosal (thiomersal)
   Preservative in vaccines, antitoxins, skin testing antigens, antiseptics, eyedrop solutions, contact lens solutions and cosmetic products such as eye make-up.

9. Sesquiterpene lactone mix
   0.1% dilution of an equal mixture of alantolactone, costunolide and dehydrocostuslactone, used in the detection of Compositae sensitivity.

10. Hydrocortisone-17-butyrate
    Used as a topical corticosteroid with anti-inflammatory properties.
    Marker for some cases of topical corticosteroid allergy.

11. 2,5 Diazolidinylurea
    Formaldehyde-releaser used as a cosmetic preservative in, e.g., lotions,
    creams, shampoos and hair gels. Known also under the trade name
    Germall II.

12. Cetylstearylalcohol
    A combination of cetyl (C 16) and stearyl (C18) alcohols 50/50 used as
    emulsifier and emollient in cosmetic lotions, creams, ointments and
    pharmaceutical preparations.

13. Toluenesulphonamide formaldehyde resin
    Modifier and adhesion promoter for film natural and synthetic resins.
    Occurs in vinyl lacquers, nitrocellulose compositions (e.g. nail lac-
    quers), PVA adhesives, acrylics.

14. Propylene glycol
    Vehicle in pharmaceutical and cosmetic bases. In food as solvent for
    colours and flavours and to prevent growth of moulds. Present in cool-
    ing fluids.

4.9
Additional Series of Patch Tests

The (extended) standard series of patch tests has some limitations. Cohorts
of allergens are present in our environment. In each patient, additional
allergens must be considered, according to the personal history; it is sometimes necessary to test with unknown products (see Sect. 7.6). In order to
improve the performance of the patch testing procedure, several research
groups have proposed additional series of patch tests, suitable in well-defined environmental and/or work exposures. Such series are available from
companies. The Chemotechnique and Trolab Hermal catalogues provide
useful information [10, 11]. The clinician must adapt his (her) choice to each
individual patient. It is beyond the scope of this book to detail all available
lists of allergens. For more information, the reader is referred to textbooks
of contact allergy, and to the above-mentioned catalogues [10, 11]. A few important lists are presented in the following sections, in alphabetical order.

4.9.1
Acrylate Series

Acrylic resins are thermoplastics formed by derivates of acrylic acid. Numerous different acrylic monomers do exist, and, as a result, a multitude of different polymers and resins are produced. Uses of acrylates are varied. The most often quoted ones are dentistry, leather finishes, adhesives, paints, printing inks and coatings, etc., but many others are described in the literature. The series presented here is certainly imperfect; nevertheless, it is useful in most cases (Table 4.5).

Table 4.5. Acrylates series (concentrations refer to petrolatum unless otherwise stated)

	Concentration (%)
1. Methyl methacrylate (MMA)	2
2. n-Butyl methacrylate (EMA)	2
3. 2-Hydroxyethyl methacrylate (2-HEMA)	2
4. 2-Hydroxypropyl methacrylate (2-HPMA)	2
5. Ethyleneglycol dimethacrylate (EGDMA)	2
6. Triethyleneglycol dimethacrylate (TREGDMA)	2
7. 1,4-Butanediol dimethacrylate (BUDMA)	2
8. Urethane dimethacrylate (UEDMA)	2
9. 2,2-Bis {4-(methacryloxy)-phenyle} propane (Bis-MA)	2
10. 2,2-Bis {4-(2hydroxy-3-methacryloxypropoxy)-phenyle} propane (Bis-GMA)	2
11. 1,6-Hexanediol diacrylate (HDDA)	0.1
12. Tetrahydrofurfuryl methacrylate	2
13. Tetraethyleneglycol dimethacrylate (TEGDMA)	2
14. N,N-Dimethylaminoethyl methacrylate	0.2
15. Ethyl cyanoacrylate	10

4.9.2
Bakers Series

This series includes several allergens encountered in bakeries and confectioneries (Table 4.6).

Table 4.6. Bakers series (concentrations refer to petrolatum unless otherwise stated)

	Concentration (%)
1. Sodium benzoate	5
2. 2-*tert*-Butyl-4 methoxyphenol	2
3. Anethole	5
4. Sorbic acid	2
5. Benzoic acid	5
6. Propionic acid	3
7. Octyl gallate	0.25
8. Dipentene (limonene)	1
9. Ammonium persulphate	2.5
10. Propyl gallate	1
11. Benzoyl peroxyde	1
12. Dodecyl gallate	0.25

4.9.3
Cosmetic Series

This series is the result of a proposal of the Belgian Contact and Environmental Dermatitis Group (BCEDG). It is not limiting (Table 4.7).

Table 4.7. Cosmetic series (concentrations refer to petrolatum unless otherwise stated)

		Concentration (%)
1.	Sodium metabisulphite	2
2.	Cetrimide	0.05 (aq.)
3.	Benzoic acid	5
4.	Sorbic acid	2
5.	Butylhydroxyanisole (BHA)	2
6.	Chlorhexidine digluconate	0.5 (aq.)
7.	Nonoxynol 9	2 (aq.)
8.	Castor oil, hydrogenated	20
9.	Phenoxyethanol	5
10.	Chloracetamide	0.2
11.	Triclosan (Irgasan DP300)	2
12.	Bronopol	0.5
13.	Cocamidopropylbetaine	1 (aq.)

4.9.4
Drug Series

Drug (or medicament) series are available. Nevertheless, it does not seem reasonable to apply such series, since drugs have been chosen at random. A precisely oriented patch test series is advised for each patient.

4.9.5
Hairdressers Series

This series includes allergens present in permanent waving formulations, permanent hair dyes, hair bleaches and preservatives (Table 4.8).

Table 4.8. Hairdressers series (concentrations refer to petrolatum unless otherwise stated)

		Concentration (%)
1.	Ammonium thioglycolate	1
2.	*p*-Aminodiphenylamine chlorhydrate	0.25
3.	*p*-Toluylenediamine	1
4.	*p*-Toluylenediamine sulphate	1
5.	o-Nitro-*p*-phenylenediamine	1
6.	3-Aminophenol	1
7.	Resorcinol	1
8.	Pyrogallol	1
9.	Glyceryl monothioglycolate (GMTG)	1
10.	Chloracetamide	0.2
11.	Cocoamidopropylbetaïne	1 (aq.)
12.	Ammonium persulphate	2.5

4.9.6
Metals Series

This short series of additional metals may be very useful in some cases (Table 4.9).

Table 4.9. Metals series (concentrations refer to petrolatum unless otherwise stated)

		Concentration (%)
1.	Potassium dicyanoaurate	0.002
2.	Sodium thiosulfatoaurate	0.5
3.	Ammonium tetrachloroplatinate	0.25
4.	Palladium chloride	1
5.	Copper sulphate	1
6.	Aluminium	As is

4.9.7
Pesticides Series

The series is not frequently used in practice (Table 4.10).

Table 4.10. Pesticides series (concentrations refer to petrolatum unless otherwise stated)

		Concentration (%)
1.	Captan	0.1
2.	Zineb (Zinc ethylene bis dithiocarbamate)	1
3.	Captafol (Difolatan)	0.1
4.	Maneb	1
5.	Folpet (Phaltan)	0.1
6.	Pyrethrum	2
7.	Benomyl	1
8.	Ziram (Zinc dimethyldithiocarbamate)	1

4.9.8
Plastics and Glues Series

Note that this series is in some way misleading, since many new allergens are regularly introduced in the technological procedures involved in the plastics and glues industry. Caution is therefore needed in its interpretation (Table 4.11).

4.9.9
Rubber Additives Series

The technology of rubber vulcanization is complex and involves the occurrence of various chemicals, some of which have a high allergenic potential (Table 4.12).

4.9.10
Textile Dyes and Finish Series

The series includes textile dyes (of the azo, anthraquinone, or nitro type) and chemicals occasionally present in textile finish (Table 4.13).

Table 4.11. Plastics and glues series (concentrations refer to petrolatum unless otherwise stated)

		Concentration (%)
1.	Hexamethylenetetramine	2
2.	Triethylenetetramine	0.5
3.	Phenylglycidylether	0.25
4.	Diethylenetriamine	1
5.	Epoxy resin cycloaliphatic	0.5
6.	Dimethylaminopropylamine	1
7.	Isophoronediamine	0.1
8.	Toluene diisocyanate (TDI)	2
9.	Diphenylmethane-4,4 diisocyanate (NDI)	2
10.	Isophorone diisocyanate (IPDI)	1
11.	1,6 Hexamethylenediisocyanate (HDI)	0.1
12.	Hydroquinone	1
13.	Dibutylphthalate	5
14.	Phenylsalicylate	1
15.	Diethylhexylphthalate (dioctylphthalate)	2
16.	2,6 Ditert-butyl-4-cresol (BHT)	2
17.	2(2-Hydroxy-5-methylphenyl) benzotriazol	1
18.	Benzoyl peroxide	1
19.	4-*tert*-Butylcatechol (PTBC)	0.25
20.	Azodiisobutyrodinitrile	1
21.	Bisphenol A	1
22.	Tricresyl phosphate	5
23.	Phenol formaldehyde resin	1
24.	Triphenyl phosphate	5
25.	Resorcinol monobenzoate	1
26.	2-Phenylindole	2
27.	2-*tert*-Butyl-4-methoxyphenol (BHA)	2
28.	Abitol	10
29.	4-*tert*-Butylphenol	1
30.	2-Monomethylol phenol	1
31.	Diphenylthiourea	1
32.	2-*n*-Octyl-4-Isothiazolin-3-one	0.1
33.	Cyclohexanone resin	1
34.	Triglycidyl isocyanurate	0.5

Table 4.12. Rubber additives series (concentrations refer to petrolatum unless otherwise stated)

		Concentration (%)
1.	Tetramethylthiuram disulphide	1
2.	Tetramethylthiuram monosulphide	1
3.	Tetraethylthiuram disulphide	1
4.	Dipentamethylenethiuram disulphide	1
5.	N-Cyclohexyl-N-phenyl-4-phenylenediamine	1
6.	N,N-Diphenyl-4-phenylenediamine	1
7.	N-Cyclohexylbenzothiazyl sulphenamide	1
8.	Dibenzothiazyl disulphide	1
9.	Morpholinyl mercaptobenzothiazole	1
10.	N,N-Diphenylguanidine	1
11.	Zinc diethyldithiocarbamate	1
12.	Zinc dibutyldithiocarbamate	1
13.	N,N-Di-beta naphtyl-4-phenylenediamine	1
14.	N-Phenyl-2-naphtylamine	1
15.	Hexamethylenetetramine	2
16.	Diphenylthiourea	1
17.	Zinc dimethyldithiocarbamate (Ziram)	1
18.	2,2,4-Trimethyl-1,2-dihydroquinoline	1
19.	Diethylthiourea	1
20.	Dibutylthiourea	1
21.	Dodecylmercaptan	0.1
22.	N-Cyclohexylthiophthalimide	1

Table 4.13. Textile dyes and finish series (concentrations refer to petrolatum unless otherwise stated)

		Concentration (%)
1.	Disperse orange 1	1
2.	Disperse orange 3	1
3.	Disperse brown 1	1
4.	Disperse red 1	1
5.	Disperse red 17	1
6.	Disperse yellow 3	1
7.	Disperse yellow 9	1
8.	Disperse blue 3	1
9.	Disperse blue 35	1
10.	Disperse blue 85	1
11.	Disperse blue 106	1
12.	Disperse blue 153	1
13.	Disperse blue 124	1
14.	*p*-Aminophenol	2
15.	Dimethylol dihydroxyethyleneurea	4.5 (aq.)
16.	Dimethyl dihydroxyethyleneurea	4.5 (aq.)
17.	Dimethylol dihydroxyethyleneurea modified	5 (aq.)
18.	Ethyleneurea, melamineformaldehyde (sorbitan sesquioleate)	5
19.	Urea formaldehyde	10
20.	Melamine formaldehyde	7

References

1. Jadassohn W (1951) A propos des tests épicutanés "dirigés" dans l'eczéma professionnel. Praxis 40:1–4
2. Foussereau J, Benezra C (1970) Les eczémas allergiques professionnels. Masson, Paris
3. Bloch B (1929) The role of idiosyncrasy and allergy in dermatology. Arch Dermatol Syphilis 19:175–197
4. Bonnevie P (1939) Aetiologie und Pathogenese der Ekzemkrankheiten. Klinische Studien über die Ursachen der Ekzeme unter besonderer Berücksichtigung des Diagnostischen Wertes der Ekzemproben. Busch, Copenhagen/Barth, Leipzig
5. Wahlberg JE (2001) Patch testing. In: Rycroft RJG, Menné T, Frosch PJ, Lepoittevin JP (eds) Textbook of contact dermatitis, 3rd edn. Springer, Berlin, p 458
6. de Groot AC, Frosch PJ (2001) Patch test concentrations and vehicles for testing contact allergens. In: Rycroft RJG, Menné T, Frosch PJ, Lepoittevin JP (eds) Textbook of contact dermatitis, 3rd edn. Springer, Berlin, p 1040
7. Hansson C, Agrup G (1993) Stability of the mercaptobenzothiazole compounds. Contact Dermatitis 28:29–34
8. Lachapelle JM, Ale SI, Freeman S, Frosch PJ, Goh CL, Hannuksela M, Hayakawa R, Maibach HI, Wahlberg JE (1997) Proposal for a revised international standard series of patch tests. Contact Dermatitis 36:121–123
9. Dooms-Goossens A, Andersen KE, Brandao FM, Bruynzeel D, Burrows D, Camarasa J, Ducombs G, Frosch P, Hannuksela M, Lachapelle JM, Lahti A, Menné T, Wahlberg JE, Wilkinson JD (1996) Corticosteroid contact allergy: EECDRG Multicentre Study. Contact Dermatitis 35:40–44
10. Chemotechnique Catalogue (2001) Chemotechnique diagnostics. Malmö, Sweden
11. Trolab® Hermal Catalogue (2001) Reinbek, Germany

Chapter 5

Photopatch Testing

J.-M. Lachapelle, S. Freeman

Photopatch testing, simply stated, is patch testing with the addition of UV radiation to induce formation of the photoallergen. Application of allergens and scoring criteria are the same as those described for plain patch testing (see Chap. 3). The only additional equipment that is necessary is an appropriate light source and opaque shielding for the period after removal of the patch test material before readings [1].

Photopatch testing is intended to detect the responsible photoallergen(s) in two clinical situations, namely, photoallergic contact dermatitis and photoallergic drug eruptions. Nevertheless, these two conditions cannot always be easily diagnosed from other dermatoses, induced and/or worsened by exposure to light, i.e. chronic actinic dermatitis (CAD), polymorphic light eruption (PLE), and other variants of photosensitivity. Therefore, some authors recommend that all photosensitive patients should be photopatch tested [1]. Photoallergic contact dermatitis (PACD) can in fact be superimposed on PLE.

The strategies for assessing the relevance of positive photopatch testing results are similar to those used for plain patch testing (see Chap. 8).

5.2
Photoallergic Contact Dermatitis

PACD is produced when sensitization occurs from the combination of skin contact with a compound together with ultraviolet light (UVL) exposure. In these cases the hapten requires UVL to be fully activated. Such pa-

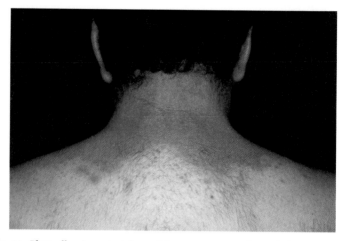

Fig. 5.1. Photoallergic contact dermatitis to a sunscreen. Covered sites are spared

tients develop a dermatitis on light-exposed sites. This typically involves the face, neck, dorsal hands, and forearms, but spares shaded sites such as the upper eyelids, submental area, and post-auricular areas (Fig. 5.1).

However, PACD has become less common because of the withdrawal from the market of many photocontact sensitizers. In the past 30 years, several notorious photoallergens were identified. Musk ambrette and 6 methyl coumarin were found to be potent photosensitizers present in fragrances. Their use has now been banned by the International Fragrance Association (IFRA). Halogenated salicylanilides and chlorinated phenols, e.g. bithionol, fenticlor and tribromosalicylanilide (TBS), were popular antiseptic and antifungal agents. These have also been withdrawn. However, it is always possible that these photoallergens may creep in from unregulated sources. They were particularly troublesome in the past as they were capable of producing persistent light reactions. In such cases the patient continued to react to UVL even after withdrawal of the contact allergen. Fortunately such problems are now rarely seen.

However, with the ever-increasing number of new products coming on the market, there is always the possibility of the appearance of new photoallergens. An important example is the increasing use of sunscreens, which are now often incorporated into cosmetic products where their use may not be so obvious. All the sunscreen chemicals which absorb UVL are capable of producing PACD. These include the *p*-aminobenzoic acid (PABA) products, the cinnamates, the benzophenones, oxybenzones and dibenzoyl methanes (Table 5.1). The reflectant sunscreens which act as a physical barrier are not photosensitizers (i.e. zinc oxide and titanium dioxide). Sunscreens are now the most common photocontact

Table 5.1. Proposed allergens for a photopatch test series (concentrations refer to petrolatum)

		Concentration (%)
A. Sunscreen series		
1	4-*tert*-Butyl-4'-methoxy-dibenzoylmethane (Parsol 1789, Eusolex 9020)	10
2	4-Aminobenzoic acid (PABA)	10
3	Homosalate	5
4	3-(4-Methylbenzyliden)camphor (Eusolex 6300)	10
5	2-Ethylhexyl-4-dimethylaminobenzoate (Eusolex 6007, Escalol 507, Octyl dimethyl-PABA)	10
6	2-Hydroxy-4-methoxybenzophenone (Eusolex 4360, Escalol 567, Oxybenzone, Benzophenone-3)	10
7	2-Ethylhexyl-4-methoxycinnamate (Parsol MCX, Escalol 557)	10
8	2-Hydroxy-methoxymethylbenzophenone (Mexenone)	10
9	2-Phenylbenzimidazol-5-sulphonic acid (Eusolex 232, Novantisol)	10
10	2-Hydroxy-4-methoxybenzophenon-5-sulphonic acid (Sulisobenzone,Uvinyl MS-40, Benzophenone 4)	10
B. Additional tests (optional, according to patient's history)		
a	Cosmetic products	As is
b	Drugs (check irritation)	10–30
c	Occupational: olaquindox	1
d	Patient's own products, as appropriate	Suitable dilution

allergens seen [2]. However, the benefits of sunscreens still greatly out-weigh the risks. Sunscreens form the basis of any photopatch test series (Table 5.1).

Another example of a photocontact allergen identified in recent years is olaquindox [3]. This is a chemotherapeutic growth-promoter used in food for pigs. It was marketed in 1975 as a 10% premix with vitamins and minerals. It forms a dusty mixture to which pig farmers are easily exposed when they add it to their pigs' food. As the work is usually outdoors it can be a potent photocontact allergen for the pig farmers. It can also produce persistent light reactors. Withdrawal of olaquindox and its substitution by an alternative growth promoter has been recommended and has already been instituted in some countries.

The non-steroidal anti-inflammatory drugs (NSAIDs) are increasing-ly used as topical preparations. These, too, are another reported source of PACD, as well as of allergic contact dermatitis, and drug photosensitiv-ity [4]. Since many of these compounds may also be used systemically, the possibility of development of systemic (photo- or non-photo) contact dermatitis, in patients topically sensitized, must always be borne in mind [5].

It must be emphasized that in CAD, there are often many positive patch tests (including the compositae plants), and they are usually of doubtful relevance. There is no convincing evidence that the compositae plants are photoallergens, although they may produce an airborne der-matitis distinct from a photosensitive dermatitis.

However, once again, when the history and the physical examination suggest the possibility of PACD, photopatch testing can in fact be super-imposed on an endogenous photosensitivity such as PLE.

5.3
Photoallergic Drug Eruptions

As explained elsewhere (see Chap. 12), the use of patch tests in some vari-eties of drug eruptions has been expanded in recent years, and more ex-perience has been gained in the field. This also applies to photopatch test-ing in photoallergic drug eruptions.

Similar principles of caution when interpreting positive and negative photopatch test results can be used in this respect [6].

The main drugs for which a positive photopatch test has been observed are the following: phenothiazines, NSAIDs, thiazides, fluoroquinolones, captopril, fenofibrate and thioureas.

5.4
Methodology of Photopatch Testing

The methodology of photopatch testing was first standardized in 1982 by the Scandinavian Photodermatology Research Group [7].

- Allergens are applied to the back in duplicate and covered by an opaque material. In addition to the photoallergens series (Table 5.1), any products which the patient uses on exposed sites, or is exposed to, should also be applied in duplicate.
- One set is removed after 24 h and irradiated with 5 J/cm² of ultraviolet A (UVA). If the patient shows signs of a persistent photosensitivity, the minimum erythema dose (MED) must first be determined. If the MED is found to be reduced to 1/2 of the MED, it is used for photopatch tests. The normal MED for UVA is over 20 J/cm².
- Both sets are removed after a further 24 h and read. In some centres, irradiation is carried out after 48 h, at the time of the first patch test reading. A second reading is carried out after a further 24–48 h.

The reactions are scored according to the standards of the International Contact Dermatitis Research Group (ICDRG). A true-positive photopatch test persists or increases between the first and the second readings. Phototoxic, i.e. false-positive reactions, are common. These are weak, macular reactions which fade in 24 h. An erythema occurring immediately after irradiation with UVA is also common. This is also a phototoxic response which fades in 24–48 h and is often seen with phenothiazines and antihistamine photopatch tests.

A product can be both a contact allergen and a photocontact allergen. To make a diagnosis of PACD, the photopatch test reaction should be greater than the patch test reaction.

5.5
Light Sources

The action spectrum for photoallergens lies in the UVA range (315–400 nm). Hence UVA is used for photopatch testing. Any artificial source of light with a broad-spectrum output of UVA is suitable for photopatch testing. A PUVA unit is suitable. If significant amounts of UVB are emitted, a window glass filter must be used, as UVB is far more erythemogenic than UVA. The energy output of the light source needs to be known and monitored at intervals.

The energy output of the light source must be known and monitored at intervals, as there may be fluctuation. The Waldmann Lichttechnik UV meter may serve as a standard monitoring device. At St. John's Institute of Dermatology, the light source is a bank of Philips TL 44D 25/09 fluorescent tubes. The Philips TLK 40 W/09 N fluorescent tube is free from UVB contamination [8].

5.6
Proposal for a Photopatch Test Series

At present, there is no standardized photopatch test series [8]. A working party of the European Society of Contact Dermatitis (ESCD) has undertaken the process of standardization, but the conclusions have not yet been published. A reasonable approach is to apply the sunscreen series (Chemotechnique) to each patient suspected of having PACD. Additional allergens can be chosen, with respect to the patient's history (Table 5.1).

References

1. Marks JG Jr, Elsner P, De Leo VA (2002) Contact and occupational dermatology, 3rd edn. Mosby, St. Louis
2. British Photodermatology Group (1997) Workshop report on photopatch testing methods and indications. Br J Dermatol 136:371–376
3. Schauder S, Schroder W, Geier J (1996) Olaquindox-induced airborne photoallergic contact dermatitis followed by transient or persistent light reactions in 15 pig breeders. Contact Dermatitis 35:344–354

4. Ophaswonge S, Maibach HI (1993) Topical nonsteroid anti-inflammatory drugs: allergic and photoallergic contact dermatitis and phototoxicity. Contact Dermatitis 29:57–64

5. Brandao F, Goossens A, Tosti A (2001) Topical drugs. In: Rycroft RJG, Menné T, Frosch PJ, Lepoittevin JP (eds) Textbook of contact dermatitis, 3rd edn. Springer, Berlin, pp 701–703

6. Gonçalo M (1998) Exploration dans les photoallergies médicamenteuses. In: Progrès en dermato-allergologie, Nancy 1998. John Libbey Eurotext Montrouge, France, pp 67–74

7. Jansén CT, Wennersten G, Rystedt I, Thune P, Brodthagen H (1982) The Scandinavian standard photopatch test procedure. Contact Dermatitis 8:155–158

8. White IR (2001) Photopatch testing. In: Rycroft RJG, Menné T, Frosch PJ, Lepoittevin JP (eds) Textbook of contact dermatitis, 3rd edn. Springer, Berlin, pp 527–537

CHAPTER 6

The Atopy Patch Test in Atopic Dermatitis

U. DARSOW, J. RING

6.1
Introduction

Atopic dermatitis (AD) is a chronic inflammatory skin disease, the diagnosis of which is made by a combination of clinical features. AD is characterized by recurrent intense pruritus and a typically age-related distribution and skin morphology [1, 2]. The role of allergy in eliciting and maintaining the eczematous skin lesions has been controversial, partially due to a lack of specificity of the classic tests for IgE-mediated hypersensitivity. Among the allergens found to be relevant in AD, aeroallergens and food allergens (in children) are most important. As therapeutical consequences of the diagnosis of an allergy are based upon avoidance strategies, the relevance of (often multiple) IgE-mediated sensitizations in patients with AD must be evaluated.

Environmental substances such as aeroallergens produce flares in some patients with AD. Also, aeroallergen avoidance, especially with regard to house dust mites, can result in marked improvement of skin lesions [3]. Patients with AD often have elevated serum levels of IgE, which may correlate with the disease severity. The hypothesis is that Langerhans' cells bind and present "immediate-type" allergens [4], which penetrate the impaired epidermal barrier in AD patients [5]. This concept is derived from studies showing IgE and IgE-binding structures on the surface of epidermal Langerhans' cells [5] together with mite allergen [6]. From atopy patch test biopsies, allergen-specific T cells have been cloned [7]. These T cells showed a characteristic TH2 (T-helper cell subpopulation) secretion pattern initially, whereas after 48 h a TH1 pattern was predominant. This same pattern is also found in chronic lesions of AD.

An epicutaneous patch test with allergens known to elicit IgE-mediated reactions and the evaluation of eczematous skin lesions after 48–72 h (Atopy Patch Test, APT) can be used as diagnostic tool in characterizing patients with aeroallergen-triggered AD. Several groups demonstrated that eczematous skin lesions can be induced in patients with AD by patch testing with aeroallergens. Patch testing of aeroallergens especially in patients with AD was first documented in 1982 by Mitchell et al. [8]. Due to variations in the applied methodology such as skin abrasion, tape stripping and sodium lauryl sulphate application for the enhancement of allergen penetration, differing percentages of positive APT results were obtained. No clear-cut correlations to skin prick test or specific IgE measurements could be obtained, and the sensitivity and specificity of experimental atopy patch tests with regard to clinical history remained unclear. We performed several studies to standardize the methods of APT on non-abraded skin and investigated the relation to clinical covariates.

6.2
Atopy Patch Test Technique

As a result of methodological studies [9–12], APTs with significant correlations to clinical parameters such as allergen-specific IgE and patient history are now performed with a technique very similar to conventional patch tests for the diagnosis of classic contact allergy. The standardization of aeroallergen APT is currently more advanced than that for food patch testing. In Europe these efforts are coordinated by the European Task Force on Atopic Dermatitis (ETFAD) with a multicentre trial. Epicutaneous tests with lyophilized allergens, e.g. from house dust mite (*Dermatophagoides pteronyssinus, D. pter.*), cat dander and grass pollen are performed with a petrolatum vehicle (including a vehicle control). Patients should be in a state of remission of their dermatitis; the patch test is applied in large Finn Chambers (12 mm) for 48 h on their back on non-abraded and uninvolved skin. We prefer to avoid any potentially irritating methods of skin barrier disruption such as tape stripping of the skin. Exclusion criteria (Table 6.1) and the possibility of contact urticaria should be considered. Non-atopic volunteers and patients suffering from allergic rhinoconjunctivitis only presented no positive APT reactions with our methods in several studies. Allergens in petrolatum elicited twice

Table 6.1. Proposed exclusion criteria for atopy patch test (APT). Most of these criteria must be confirmed by further clinical studies

Antihistamines except astemizole	1 week
Systemic steroids	4 weeks
Topical steroids (test area)	1 week
UV-radiation	1 week
Acute eczema flare	3 weeks

as many APT reactions as allergens in a hydrophilic vehicle. Thirty-six percent of patients reacted to house dust mite *D. pter.*, 22% to cat dander, and 16% to grass pollen. High allergen-specific IgE in serum is not a prerequisite for a positive APT, but 62% of patients with *D. pter.*-positive APT showed a corresponding positive skin prick test and 77% showed a corresponding elevated level of specific IgE. In other allergens, the concordance was even higher. Allergen concentrations of 500, 3,000, 5,000, and 10,000 PNU (protein nitrogen units)/g in petrolatum were comparatively used in 57 patients [11]. In this study, the percentage of patients with clear-cut positive reactions was significantly higher in subjects with eczematous skin lesions in air-exposed areas (69%), compared to those without this predictive pattern (39%; p=0.02). In the first group, the maximum reactivity was nearly reached with 5,000 PNU/g. The data from a randomized, double-blind multicentre trial involving 253 adult patients and 30

Table 6.2. Comparison of biological and PNU-based standardization of APT preparations: comparable concordance of APT with clinical allergen-specific history[a]

Standardization	7,000 PNU/g		200 IR/g	
Corresponding history	Yes	No	Yes	No
Dermatophagoides pteronyssinus	25	25	31	19
Cat dander	36	14	37	13
Grass pollen	39	11	39	11
Birch pollen	41	9	38	12
Total (%)	71	29	73	27

PNU, protein nitrogen units; IR, index reactif (biological unit).
[a] 400 APTs in 50 patients with atopic dermatitis.

children with atopic eczema were used to calculate a suitable APT allergen dosage [9–12]. Adults were tested with four concentrations, 3,000 to 10,000 PNU/g of *D. pter.*, cat dander, grass pollen, and (in two study centres only; *n*=88) with birch and mugwort pollen. A dose response for the APT could be obtained by McNemar statistics comparing with only questionable, only erythematous, or irritative reactions. The optimal allergen doses are in the range of 5,000–7,000 PNU/g. Simultaneously tested, the allergen doses of 7,000 PNU/g and 200 IR/g (biological unit; Index Réactif) of the most important aeroallergens in Europe showed comparable concordance with the patients' history, suggesting clinical relevance in another study on 50 patients with AD (Table 6.2).

6.3
Atopy Patch Test Reading

APT reactions are read after 48 and 72 h. Most reactions are seen after 48 h, sometimes with decrescendo to 72 h. With our methods, only very few reactions were seen as early as 24 h, but after tape stripping followed by allergen application there are more early reactions visible. APT was shown to give clinically relevant results with the ICDRG reading key for conventional patch testing [12, 13]. Consensus meetings of most groups performing APT for clinical use in Europe were held in Munich on April 11, 1997 and June 30, 1998. One result of these meetings was a consensus APT reading key for describing the intensity of APT reactions (Table 6.3). This key has more options to describe the different morphology of positive APT reactions. It is currently used in a multicentre trial in six Euro-

Table 6.3. APT reaction grading key [European Task Force on Atopic Dermatitis (ETFAD) consensus], 11 April 1997 and 30 June 1998

–	Negative
?	Only erythema, questionable
+	Erythema, infiltration
++	Erythema, few papules (up to 3)
+++	Erythema, papules from 4 to many
++++	Erythema, many or spreading papules
+++++	Erythema, vesicles

pean countries. A more important point in our opinion is to distinguish clear-cut positive reactions from negative or questionable ones, since only reactions showing papules or at least some degree of infiltration seem to be of clinical relevance.

6.4
Atopy Patch Test Relevance, Patient Subgroups and Pitfalls

To date, no "gold standard" of provocation for allergy diagnosis in AD exists. Thus, the history of allergen-specific exacerbation may be used as a parameter for clinical relevance. The validity of the APT was investigated with regard to the clinically known phenomenon of "summer eruption" of AD[13]. Seventy-nine patients were tested with 10,000 PNU/g grass pollen allergen mixture in petrolatum and simultaneously with 10 mg dry, unprocessed pollen of *Dactylis glomerata* grass. The APT results were compared with history, skin prick tests and specific corresponding IgE and the eczema pattern. This study showed significantly higher frequencies of positive APT reactions (with both methods used) in patients with a corresponding history of exacerbation of skin lesions during the grass pollen season of the previous year, or in direct contact with grass (75% with positive APT). Patients without this history showed significantly lower APT reactivity (16% with positive APT; $p<0.001$). Depending on the APT procedure, the sensitivity referred to history of exacerbations during grass pollen season was 0.67–0.75, and the specificity was 0.84–0.90. The APT specificity exceeded the specificity of the classic tests of IgE-mediated hypersensitivity, which was 0.33 for skin prick test and radioallergosorbent test (RAST). On the other hand, the sensitivity of the classical methods was higher (0.92 for RAST, and 1.0 for skin prick test). The results of unprocessed pollen leading to eczematous lesions on non-pretreated skin of AD patients with good correlation to history demonstrates that pollen may be involved in eczema flares in some patients. In the multicentre study with five aeroallergens, 10%–52% of patients reported previous eczema flares after contact with at least one of the allergens. Again, APT results were significantly correlated with history, skin prick test and specific corresponding IgE for *D. pter.*, cat dander and grass pollen ($p<0.001$). Sensitivity and specificity of the APT were calculated for every allergen with regard to the corresponding history of eczema flares (Table 6.4) [12].

Table 6.4. Sensitivity and specificity of different diagnostic methods regarding patient history in 253 patients with AD[a] (From [12])

Test	Sensitivity[b]	Specificity[b]
Skin prick	69%–82%	44%–52%
Specific IgE	65%–94%	42%–64%
APT	42%–56%	69%–92%

[a] Allergens: house dust mite *Dermatophagoides pteronyssinus*, cat dander, grass pollen. APT shows a higher specificity, but lower sensitivity compared with skin prick test and measurement of specific IgE.
[b] Referring to predictive history of eczema exacerbations in pollen season or in direct contact with allergen, excluding questionable cases, depending on allergen.

The APT with aeroallergens may provide an important diagnostic tool, as has been shown in two patient subgroups. In patients with an air-exposed eczema distribution pattern, positive APT reactions occurred at lower allergen doses compared with other patients with AD. Patients with an aeroallergen-specific history had significantly more positive APT reactions. The lower sensitivity but higher specificity of the APT compared to skin prick test or RAST favours the notion that the classical tests may have some value as screening tests, and specificity may be added by the APT. The APT does not replace the classical methods of diagnosis of IgE-mediated allergy. Questions remain open concerning the clinical relevance of positive APT results in patients with a negative history and discordant negative skin prick tests or RAST, since no gold standard exists for the provocation of eczematous skin lesions in aeroallergen-triggered AD. These questions may only be answered by conducting controlled studies using specific provocation and elimination procedures in patients with positive and negative APT results. However, this does not argue against the clinical use by dermato-allergists at this time point, since one must keep in mind that in many classic contact allergens the standardization and evaluation efforts have been less systematic. Still, these allergens are used for routine diagnosis in patch test clinics. Appropriate allergen-specific avoidance strategies are recommended in patients showing positive APT reactions. The diagnostic validity of the APT in routine diagnosis of aeroallergen-triggered atopic eczema will be investigated in further controlled studies.

Problems such as irrelevant positive or spreading APT reactions may occur in patients undergoing an APT during an eczema flare, or if methods of abrasion of the stratum corneum are used. The issue of pharmacological influence on the APT still holds many unanswered questions. As the standardization of the high-molecular-weight allergens has some specific problems, a commercial provider of test substances with reproducible quality and major allergen content is desirable. However, to date such allergen preparations are not easily available. Even more problems with allergen standardization are known for food APTs. APTs should be applied and read by dermato-allergists.

References

1. Rajka G (1989) Essential aspects of atopic dermatitis. Springer, Berlin Heidelberg New York
2. Ring J (1991) Angewandte Allergologie, 2. Aufl. MMV Medizin Verlag, Munich
3. Tan B, Weald D, Strickland I, Friedman P (1996) Double-blind controlled trial of effect of housedust-mite allergen avoidance on atopic dermatitis. Lancet 347:15–18
4. Maurer D, Ebner C, Reininger B, Fiebiger E, Kraft D, Kinet JP, Stingl G (1995) The high affinity IgE receptor mediates IgE-dependent allergen presentation. J Immunol 154:6285–90
5. Bieber T (1994) FCeRI on human Langerhans cells: a receptor in search of new functions. Immunol Today 15:52–53
6. Tanaka Y, Anan S, Yoshida H (1990) Immunohistochemical studies in mite antigen-induced patch test sites in atopic dermatitis. J Derm Science 1:361–368
7. van Reijsen FC, Bruijnzeel-Koomen CAFM, Kalthoff FS, Maggi E, Romagnani S, Westland JKT, Mudde GC (1992) Skin-derived aeroallergen-specific T-cell clones of TH2 phenotype in patients with atopic dermatitis. J Allergy Clin Immunol 90:184–192
8. Mitchell E, Chapman M, Pope F, Crow J, Jouhal S, Platts-Mills T (1982) Basophils in allergen-induced patch test sites in atopic dermatitis. Lancet 1: 127–130
9. Darsow U, Vieluf D, Berg B, Berger J, Busse A, Czech W, Heese A, Heidelbach U, Peters KP, Przybilla B, Richter G, Rueff F, Werfel T, Wistokat-Wülfing A, Ring J (1999) Dose response study of atopy patch test in children with atopic eczema. Pediatr Asthma Allergy Immunol 13:115–122
10. Darsow U, Vieluf D, Ring J (1995) Atopy patch test with different vehicles and allergen concentrations – an approach to standardization. J Allergy Clin Immunol 95:677–684

11. Darsow U, Vieluf D, Ring J (1996) The atopy patch test: an increased rate of reactivity in patients who have an air-exposed pattern of atopic eczema. Br J Dermatol 135:182–186

12. Darsow U, Vieluf D, Ring J for the APT study group. (1999) Evaluating the relevance of aeroallergen sensitization in atopic eczema using the tool "atopy patch test": a randomized, double-blind multicenter study. J Am Acad Dermatol 40:187–193

13. Darsow U, Behrendt H, Ring J (1997) Gramineae pollen as trigger factors of atopic eczema: evaluation of diagnostic measures using the atopy patch test. Br J Dermatol 137:201–207

CHAPTER 7

Additional Testing Procedures

J.-M. LACHAPELLE, H. I. MAIBACH

Patch testing remains the milestone of testing procedures in the diagnosis of allergic contact dermatitis and related diseases, in which a delayed-type (type IV) hypersensitivity is suspected (see Chap. 2). As explained in Chaps. 3–6, the technique has its own limitations and cannot by itself solve all situations encountered in environmental dermatology. Fortunately, patch testing has some undisputed "allies" to improve and prolong its performance. These additional testing procedures are discussed in the following sections.

7.1
Stripping Test

The stripping test, proposed by Spier [1], is a variant of patch testing. It consists of "stripping" the stratum corneum before applying the allergens in the usual way. The aim of the technique is to remove most layers of the stratum corneum and consequently to suppress the skin barrier. This technique is theoretically useful for allergens with a poor penetration through the skin, e.g. neomycin. It is easily carried out by stripping the skin 8 to 12 times with cellophane tape. Its main drawback is the fact that it provokes by itself skin irritation [2] that interferes at reading; nevertheless, it can be performed in well-defined conditions parallel to conventional patch testing. Reading of results needs caution and expertise.

7.2
Open Test

The open test means that a product, as is or dissolved in water or some solvent (e.g. ethanol, acetone, methylethylketone, etc.) is dropped onto the skin and allowed to spread freely. No occlusion is used. The usual test site is the volar forearm, and the surface of spreading is usually limited to 5×5 cm.

An open test is recommended as the first step when testing poorly defined or unknown substances or products, such as those brought by the patient (paints, glues, oils, cleansing agents, etc.). Readings are similar to those adopted for conventional patch testing (see Sect. 3.8). A negative open test does not preclude that allergy is not present, since it can be explained by insufficient penetration. With unknown substances, it indicates that one may go on with an occlusive patch test.

Another application of the open test is to "trap" eventual immediate (urticarial) reactions from well-known allergens, such as balsam of Peru or cinnamic aldehyde (see Sect. 3.7). The technique to be applied is similar to that described above.

7.3
Semi-Open Test

The semi-open test is an interesting variant of the open test, following the same principle of non-occlusion. The only difference from the open test is that the products, applied on the skin, are covered by a non-occlusive tape (e.g. Micropore, Fixomull) when they have dried off (about 5–10 min).

The semi-open test is thus "half-way between" open testing and conventional patch testing, and is particularly useful when testing is carried out with industrial and/or domestic products. Therefore, it is extensively used in some countries, mainly in units of occupational dermatology. Various sites can be used, such as the upper back, the extensor aspect of the arm, or the volar aspect of the forearm.

Its main advantage compared to conventional patch testing is avoidance (or reduction) of skin irritation when unknown products are applied onto the skin. It is therefore easier to make the distinction between contact allergy and irritation, but false-negative reactions frequently occur, due to insufficient penetration of products.

7.4
Repeated Open Application Test

The repeated open application test (ROAT) was standardized by Hannuk-sela and Salo [3]. Test substances, either commercial products, as is, or special test substances (e.g. patch test allergens) are applied twice daily for 7 days to the outer aspect of the upper arm, antecubital fossa or back skin (scapular area). The size of the test area is not crucial: a positive result may appear on a 1×1-cm area 1–2 days later than on a larger area. The amount of test substance should be approximately 0.1 ml to a 5×5-cm area and 0.5 ml to a 10×10-cm area [4, 5]. A positive-response eczematous dermatitis usually appears on days 2–4, but it is recommended to extend the applications beyond 7 days so as not to miss late-appearing reactions. It is our experience that reactions (as late as 20 days, i.e. 40 applications) may occur, for example with scented cosmetics (such as deodorants, creams, lotions, etc.). It is worthwhile to test at the three sites concomitantly, since one test area can react in an unpredictable way sooner than the two others. The patient is asked to stop the application of the test substance(s) when he or she notices a reaction [3]. The clinical features of positive ROAT reactions may be surprising for the dermatologist, compared to those observed in conventional patch testing.

Erythema (diffuse or spotted) and follicular elevations looking like tiny papules are commonly observed. When these symptoms appear after the first applications, irritation cannot be ruled out, and similar applications in control subjects are needed. Oedematous and/or vesicular reactions are rare (Fig. 7.1). Therefore, the technique requires correct interpretation. When carefully conducted, it provides good information and is particularly useful for comparative studies (e.g. the application of a scented cosmetic product on the three sites of the left side, compared with the application of the same product, but unscented on the right side). A refined scheme for scoring of ROAT reactions was presented recently [6].

The value of ROAT has been verified in cases with positive, negative or questionable reactions at initial patch testing and in animal studies.

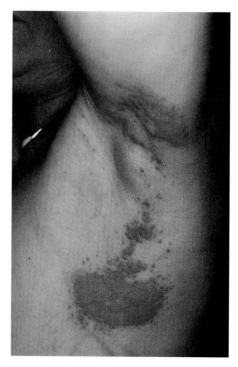

Fig. 7.1. ROAT test to a deodorant stick. Positive reaction after three applications

In essence, the provocative use test (PUT) can be considered similar (with some variants) to the ROAT test. The latter has gained international agreement.

7.5
Testing Procedures with Unknown Substances

"Wild" uncontrolled testing with totally unknown products is prohibited. Necrosis, scarring, keloids, pigmentation, depigmentation and any other complications listed earlier (see Sect. 3.14) can appear, and the dermatologist may be accused of malpractice.

7.5.1
Strategy

When patients bring suspected products or materials from their (work) environment, we recommend that adequate product safety data sheets, lists of ingredients, etc., are requested from the manufacturer so that a general impression of the product, ingredients, concentrations and intended use, can be formed. There are usually one or two ingredients that are of interest as suspected allergens, while the rest are well-known substances of proven innocuousness and/or known irritancy for which detailed information is available. For substances or products where skin contact is unintentional and the dermatitis is a result of misuse or accident, detailed information from the manufacturer is required before any tests are initiated [7].

7.5.2
Steps Required Prior to Any Testing Procedure

The next step is to look for the suspected allergens. If they are available from suppliers of patch test allergens, one can rely on the choice of vehicle and concentration. If one suspects that impurities or contaminants caused the dermatitis, this can only be discovered via samples of the ingredient from the manufacturer.

If it is an entirely new substance, where no data on toxicity are available, the patient and the dermatologist must decide how to find an optimal test concentration and vehicle, and must discuss the risk of complications. To minimize the risk, one can start with an open test and, if this is negative, continue with occlusive patch testing. Most allergens are tested in the concentration range 0.01%–10%, and we usually start with the lowest and raise the concentration when the preceding test is negative. A practical method is to apply 0.01% and 0.1% for 1 day in a region where the patient can easily remove the patch her- or himself (upper back or upper arm). If severe stinging of burning occurs, the patient should be instructed to remove the patch immediately. If the test is negative, the concentration can be raised to 1%. Occasionally, the likely irritant or sensitization potential of a chemical may be such that starting with concentrations of 0.001% and 0.01% is advisable, increasing to 0.1% if negative. An alternative is to start with a higher concentration, but with reduced exposure time (5 h), but this procedure is not sufficiently standardized.

An important check point is the pH of the product to be tested. It is unwise to test with a product whose pH is below 4 or above 9.

If the patient's test is positive, the clinician must demonstrate in unexposed controls that the actual test preparation is non-irritant. Otherwise the observed reaction in the particular patient does not prove allergenicity.

When testing products brought by the patient, it is essential to use samples from the actual batch to which the patient was exposed, but also when testing, for example, cutting fluids, unused products must be tested for comparison. When testing with dilutions, one runs the risk of overlooking true allergens by using over-diluted materials.

7.5.3
Testing Procedures with Solid Products and Extracts

When a solid product is suspected (e.g. textiles, rubber, plants, wood, paper), this can usually be applied as is. Rycroft [8] recommends that the material be tested as wafer-thin, regular-sided, smooth sheets (e.g. rubber) or as finely divided particulates (e.g. woods). Plants and woods and their extracts constitute special problems, due to variations in the quantity of allergens produced and their availability on the surface. Extracts for testing can be obtained by placing the product or sample in water, synthetic sweat, ethanol, acetone or ether, and heating to 40°–50°C. False reactions to non-standardized patch tests have been reviewed by Rycroft [8].

When patch testing with solid materials, a classic unwanted reaction is the pressure effect (see Sect. 3.14).

7.5.4
Testing Procedures with Cosmetics and Other Related Products

For most products with intended use on normal or damaged skin (e.g. cosmetics, skin care products, soaps, shampoos, detergents, topical medicaments), detailed predictive testing and clinical and consumer trials have been performed. The results can usually be obtained from the manufacturer. For this category of products, open tests (see Sect. 7.2), semi-open tests (see Sect. 7.3) and ROAT tests (see Sect. 7.4) probably give more information on the pathogenesis of the patient's dermatitis than an occlusive patch test does. Suggestions on concentrations and vehicles can be found in textbooks.

7.6
Oral Provocation Test (Oral Challenge)

The oral provocative test is rarely conducted in the field of allergic contact dermatitis. It has been mainly used in cases of recurrent vesicular palmar eczema (pompholyx), in which systemic administration of allergens is considered significant in provoking recurrences of the disease. Nickel is the most often incriminated culprit [9].

The assumption that there is an association between nickel allergy and recurrent vesicular hand eczema is supported by several trials of placebo-controlled oral challenge with doses of nickel ranging from 0.5 to 5.6 mg. These studies indicate that an oral dose of nickel may reactivate vesicular hand eczema in nickel-sensitive patients and that the response is dose-dependent. A dose of 0.5 mg nickel will reactivate vesicular hand eczema in only a small proportion of nickel-sensitive patients. Oral challenge with 2.5 mg nickel will cause a flare of dermatitis in approximately 50% of such patients, and a majority of nickel-sensitive patients will experience a flare-up reaction after a dose of 5.6 mg nickel [10]. Foods rich in nickel content may cause flares of vesicular hand eczema.

Cobalt and chromates have also been suspected, but oral challenge with these metals is not of common use.

Other investigations are related to balsam of Peru and spices. These are sparse. Veien et al. [11] challenged 17 balsam-sensitive patients with 1 g balsam of Peru. Four of four patients with recurrent pompholyx had flare-up reactions after oral challenge with balsam but not after challenge with a placebo. Dooms-Goossens et al. [12] studied reactions to spices and described three patients who had pompholyx that flared after ingestion of various spices.

7.7
Spot Tests

Spot tests can be used to demonstrate both inorganic and organic compounds in several items [13]. A specific reagent may react with a specific substance to give a specific colour and thus indicate the occurrence of the specific substance. A few spot tests can be used routinely by dermatologists.

7.7.1
Dimethylglyoxime Test for Nickel

Nickel is most commonly detected by using the dimethylglyoxime test. A few drops each of dimethylglyoxime 1% in ethanol and ammonium hydroxide 10% in water are applied to a cotton-tipped applicator, which is rubbed against the metal object to be investigated. Dimethylglyoxime reacts with nickel ions in the presence of ammonia, giving a red salt. Coins known to contain nickel can be used to test the reagent and to observe the pink colour. The solutions can also be applied directly on the metallic objects. Chemotechnique has developed a nickel spot test that consists of an ammoniacal solution of dimethylglyoxime (thus, only one solution is used). The test detects free nickel down to a limit of 10 ppm. The sensitivity of the test can be enhanced by pretreatment of the surface of the object with a solution of synthetic sweat and by heating. The method is very simple and can be used by dermatologists and nickel-allergic patients to detect nickel release from various metallic objects (Fig. 7.2).

7.7.2
Other Spot Tests

Other spot tests are available [13], mainly for detection of chromates and formaldehyde.

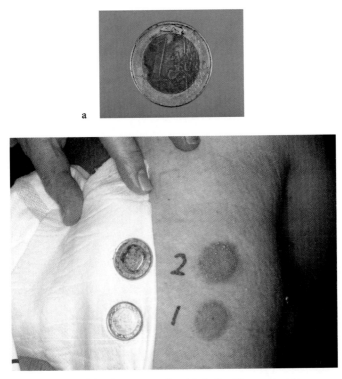

Fig. 7.2. a, b. Dimethylglyoxime spot test for nickel. **a** Positive spot test. One-euro coin. **b** Positive patch test to one- and two-euro coins in a patient sensitized to nickel

7.8
Chemical Analysis

To detect the presence of allergens in products or items brought by patients, chemical analysis can be performed in specialized laboratories. There are many available techniques; these include thin-layer chromatography, gas chromatography, atomic absorption spectrophotometry, UV-VIS spectrophotometry, infrared spectrophotometry, mass spectrometry and nuclear magnetic resonance spectroscopy [13].

References

1. Spier HW, Sixt I (1955) Untersuchungen über die Abhängigkeit des Ausfalles der Ekzem Lappchenprobes van der Hornschichtdieke (Quantitativer Abrisss-Epicutantest). Hautarzt 6:152–159
2. Schaefer H, Redelmeier TE (1996) Skin barrier. Principles of percutaneous absorption. Karger, Basel, p 172
3. Hannuksela M, Salo H (1986) The repeated open application test (ROAT). Contact Dermatitis 14:221–227
4. Hannuksela M (1991) Sensitivity of various skin sites in the repeated open application test. Am J Contact Dermatitis 2:102–104
5. Hannuksela A, Niinimäki A, Hannuksela M (1993) Size of the test area does not affect the result of the repeated open application test. Contact Dermatitis 28:299–300
6. Johansen JD, Bruze M, Andersen KE, Frosch PJ, Dreier B, White IR, Rastogi S, Lepoittevin JP, Menné T (1998) The repeated open application test: Suggestions for a scale of evaluation. Contact Dermatitis 39:95–96
7. Wahlberg JE (2001) Patch testing. In: Rycroft RJG, Menné T, Frosch PJ, Lepoittevin JP (eds) Textbook of contact dermatitis, 3rd edn. Springer, Berlin, pp 462–463
8. Rycroft RJG (1986) False reactions to nonstandard patch tests. Semin Dermatol 5:225–230
9. Veien NK, Menné T (2000) Acute and recurrent vesicular hand dermatitis (pompholyx). In: Menné T, Maibach HI (eds) Hand eczema, 2nd edn. CRC Press, Boca Raton, pp 147–164
10. Veien NK, Hattel T, Justesen O, Nørholm A (1987) Oral challenge with nickel and cobalt in patients with positive patch tests to nickel and/or cobalt. Acta Derm Venereol 67:321–325
11. Veien NK, Hattel T, Justesen O, Nørholm A (1985) Oral challenge with balsam of Peru. Contact Dermatitis 12:104–107
12. Dooms-Goossens A, Dubelloy R, Degreef H (1990) Contact and systemic contact-type dermatitis to spices. Contact Dermatitis 8:89–92
13. Gruvberger B, Bruze M, Fregert S (2001) Spot tests and chemical analyses for allergen evaluation. In: Rycroft RJG, Menné T, Frosch PJ, Lepoittevin JP (eds) Textbook of contact dermatitis, 3rd edn. Springer, Berlin, pp 495–510

CHAPTER 8

Clinical Relevance of Patch Test Reactions

J.-M. LACHAPELLE, I. ALE, H. I. MAIBACH

8.1
Introduction

Reading patch test results cannot be limited to scoring as positive or negative. Scoring in itself has no meaning if it is not linked in some way with the medical history of the patient. In other words, a positive patch test (and to some extent a negative patch test) has no interest if it is not labelled as relevant or non-relevant. Incidentally, this concept is also valid for all laboratory investigations.

8.2
General Principles

To diagnose allergic contact dermatitis, two significant steps should be considered:

1. Demonstrating the existence of contact allergy to one or several allergens
2. Demonstrating their clinical relevance

The first step is fulfilled when a positive patch test reaction deemed to reveal the presence of a genuine contact hypersensitivity is obtained. This involves assessing the morphology of the reaction and deciding whether it represents a true-positive allergic reaction as opposed to a false-positive one. Accurate reading and interpretation of patch test reactions are difficult tasks. Different variables, i.e. type of patch test system, sources of patch test allergens, amount of allergen applied, criteria of patient's selection, application and reading times, skin area, and variations in biological responsiveness, may influence the test result [1]. Another notorious disadvantage of patch testing is that reading is eminently subjective, based on inspection and palpation of the test sites. Even if the International Contact Dermatitis Research Group (ICDRG) criteria concerning a uniform scoring system for patch test readings and a quantitative scale for positive reactions (from + to +++) are generally accepted, the exact definition of the morphological criteria of this scale is still not uniform, and there are also slight variations in the categorization between the different research groups [2].

After arriving – not without difficulty – at an interpretation indicating contact sensitivity to a defined allergen, there is still one more issue to overcome, i.e. demonstrating its relevance to the clinical situation. We will not herein consider the assessment of the relevance of the negative reactions, undoubtedly of significance to address the issue of false-negative responses. Moreover, doubtful reactions may be clinically relevant according to undeniable clinical criteria or follow-up testing. It could be worthwhile to ascertain whether doubtful (?) or weak (+) patch test reactions yield a significantly different relevance score than stronger and presumably more reliable positive patch test reactions.

Assessing the relevance of a positive patch test reaction is complex and involves many confounding factors. Evaluating the relevance of a reaction is the most difficult and intricate part of the patch test procedure, and is a challenge to both dermatologist and patient. The dermatologist's skill, experience and curiosity are crucial factors. Little or no data on clinical relevance are provided in many clinical studies. Moreover, there is not a consensus as to the definition of clinical relevance, how it should be scored, and how it should be assessed [3].

8.3
Past and Current Relevance

According to the ICDRG criteria, we consider that a positive patch test reaction is "relevant" if the allergen is traced. If the source of a positive patch test is not traced, we consider it an "unexplained positive". We use the term "current" or "present" relevance if the positive patch test putatively explains the patient's present dermatitis. Similarly, when the positive patch test explains a past clinical disease, not directly related to the current symptoms, we refer to this as past relevance. However, recurrent but discontinuous contact with an allergen can occur in some patients, making it difficult to discriminate between current and past relevance [4].

8.4
Scoring System

A modified relevance scoring system was proposed by Lachapelle [4] (Tables 8.1, 8.2) for categorizing present and past relevance of positive patch tests reactions. The system codifies relevance scores from 0 to 3: 0=not traced, 1=doubtful, 2=possible, and 3=likely. Therefore, 16 combinations can be pondered for each individual case. The NACDG utilizes a

Table 8.1. The relevance scoring system of positive patch test reactions (from [4])

Past relevance (PR)	
PR 0	Not traced
PR 1	Doubtful
PR 2	Possible
PR 3	Likely
Current relevance (CR)	
CR 0	Not traced
CR 1	Doubtful
CR 2	Possible
CR 3	Likely

Table 8.2. Concomitant recording of past relevance (PR) and current relevance (CR) scores of positive patch test reactions: the 16 potential combinations (from [4])

PR0 CR3	PR0 CR2
PR1 CR3	PR1 CR2
PR2 CR3	PR2 CR2
PR3 CR3	PR3 CR2
PR0 CR1	PR0 CR0
PR1 CR1	PR1 CR0
PR2 CR1	PR2 CR0
PR3 CR1	PR3 CR0

similar scoring system using the terms "relevance possible", "relevance probable" and "relevance definite" [5].

Our goal in assessing relevance is to ascertain the putative responsibility of a particular allergen to the clinical circumstance. In this sense, the exposure to the incriminated allergen may explain the dermatitis entirely, i.e. "complete relevance"; but dermatitis with a multifactorial background frequently occurs. Contact sensitization may complicate dermatitis with an endogenous background, and other exogenous factors, such as irritants, may also play a significant role. Hence, we use the term "partial relevance" when the patch test-positive allergen contributed to or aggravated the dermatitis. It may be complicated, and often unattainable, to assess the relative influence of the different exogenous and endogenous factors on a given case of dermatitis.

8.5
Strategies

Therefore, determining the relevance of a positive patch test reaction principally relies upon the judicious interpretation of the clinical facts [6]. An allergen is clinically relevant if:

1. We can establish the existence of an exposure
2. The patient's dermatitis is explainable (totally or partially) with regard to that exposure

Establishing exposure involves appropriate knowledge of the patient's chemical environment and perseverance in pursuing lines of investigation. Relevance can be defined as the capability of an information retrieval system to select and redeem data appropriate to a patient's need [4].

8.5.1
Clinical History

The assessment starts with a comprehensive clinical history (Table 8.3). The patient should be questioned about occupational exposure, homework, and hobbies. Use of skin care products, topical medications and protective measures should be covered. Emphasis should be made on pos-

Table 8.3. Clinical data for the assessment of relevance

1.	History of exposure to the sensitizer (present or past), specially seeking for intolerance

    Occupational exposure
        Complete job description and materials
        Personal protective measures at work (gloves, masks, barrier creams)
        Other materials present in the working environment

    Non-occupational exposure
    Homework, hobbies
    Skin care products, nail and hair products, fragrances
    Pharmaceutical products (by prescription and over the counter)
    Personal protective measures. Use of gloves, detergents, etc.
    Jewellery and clothing

    Indirect contact (skin care and other products of partner, fomites, etc.)

    Seasonal related contact (plants and other environmental agents)

    Photoexposure

    Type of exposure: dose, frequency, site

    Environmental conditions: humidity, temperature, occlusion, vapours, powders, mechanical trauma, friction, etc.

2. Clinical characteristics of the present dermatitis
    Time of onset and characteristics of the initial lesions
    Dermatitis area corresponding to the exposure site
    Some morphologies suggest specific allergens
    Clinical course (caused or aggravated by the exposure)
    Time relationship to work. Effect of holidays and time-off work

3. History of previous dermatitis and other clinical events
    Past exogenous dermatitis with similar or different characteristics
    Previous patch testing
    Other endogenous skin diseases (psoriasis, atopic dermatitis, stasis, etc.)

4. Personal and family atopy and history of other family skin diseases

sible exposures to the responsible environmental allergen or chemically related substances. Frequently it proves worthwhile to inform the patient in writing about the allergen producing the reaction, different names under which it is present, sources of exposure and chemical relatives. A complete review of the patient's history should provide insight into differentiating allergic contact dermatitis from other exogenous or endogenous dermatitis. This is crucial when dealing with multifactorial dermatitis.

8.5.2
Environmental Evaluation

Historical data should be confirmed and supplemented by a rigorous environmental evaluation including research into the composition of products to which the patient has been exposed [7]. Identifying all possible sources of exposure in the subject's environment is an indispensable yet troublesome procedure involving many qualitative and quantitative estimations (Table 8.4). The intrinsic allergenic potential of the suspected agent as well as other physicochemical properties should be considered.

Table 8.4. Evaluation of exposure for the assessment of relevance

1.	Clinical history (looking for all possible sources of exposure)
2.	Workplace visit
3.	Assessment of intrinsic sensitization potential of the substance Data from predictive tests Data from epidemiological studies Structure/activity analysis
4.	Additional physicochemical properties of the substance Solvent properties, hygroscopicity, substantivity, wash and rub resistance to removal, etc.
5.	Assessment of exposure parameters Route of exposure Specific site of contact and surface area Dose Duration Frequency (periodicity) of exposure Simultaneous exposure factors: humidity, occlusion, temperature, mechanical trauma
6.	Look for cross-reacting and concomitant allergens
7.	Information from "lists" of allergens, databases, product's manufacturer, etc.
8.	Chemical analysis of suspected products

In addition, other exposure characteristics such as route of exposure, specific cutaneous site of contact, total contact area, dose, duration and frequency of exposure are crucial factors in both the sensitization and elicitation phases of allergic contact dermatitis. Relevance scores and accuracy of the assessment are significantly improved by a comprehensive knowledge of the patient's chemical environment. Visiting the patient's workplace enables the physician to obtain a comprehensive picture of the real conditions at the working environment, bringing many details into clinical significance. Useful information about sources of allergens may be obtained from textbooks, "lists" of allergens, material safety data sheets and manufacturers. Sometimes, chemical analysis of the supposedly causative product(s) is necessary. Simple qualitative chemical spot tests performed by the clinician may orient the laboratory work [8]. Specialized techniques for allergen isolation and quantitative microanalysis are required in many cases. In some circumstances it may be difficult to substantiate the presence of the allergen in the patient's environment. This may be due to the complexity in detecting certain allergens or to insufficient knowledge about the composition of different products. As a consequence, the relevance scores for different allergens will vary; the easier the identification of the source of an allergen, the higher the relevance scores. Absolute proof of relevance is often unattainable, as it is frequently not known whether suspected products actually contain the implicated allergen in sufficient amount to elicit the dermatitis.

8.5.3
Further Correlations

The history of exposure to the sensitizer is essential, but not sufficient to establish the clinical relevance. To ascertain whether the exposure is relevant to the clinical dermatitis, the following factors should be considered:

1. Existence of a temporal relationship between the exposure and the clinical course of the dermatitis
2. Correspondence between the exposure and the clinical pattern (anatomical distribution) of the dermatitis

When actually present, these two conditions provide crucial diagnostic clues. Different confounding factors should be considered, i.e. the contact with the allergen is not direct (e.g. airborne, ectopic, or connubial dermatitis); the clinical pattern of the dermatitis is non-specific or has been modified (e.g. previous treatment, secondary infection, etc.); the dermatitis is multifactorial and factors other than contact allergy must also be considered as a cause (e.g. irritation, atopy, stasis, eczematous psoriasis) [6]. Often the clinical situation is intricate, demanding a systematic and critical approach.

8.6
Additional Investigations

Additional tests may prove valuable in establishing a definite causative relationship (Table 8.5). Tests with products to which the patients refer exposure and which supposedly contain the putative allergen should be performed. Patch testing with the unmodified product frequently produces negative results. This may be due to:

Table 8.5. Testing procedures for the assessment of relevance

1.	Testing with the suspected allergen(s)
	 Sequential patch testing
	 Repeated open application test (ROAT) or provocative use test (PUT)
	   On normal skin
	   On slightly damaged or previously dermatitic skin

2.	Testing with products suspected to contain the responsible allergen Patch testing (using suitable vehicle and appropriate concentration, frequently starting with highly diluted substances) ROAT (similar as stated above, using proper vehicle and adequate concentration) Use test (typical product use) Testing in normal controls (if necessary)
3.	Testing with product's extracts Similar to 2. Testing with products suspected to contain the responsible allergen
4.	Testing with cross-reacting allergens and products suspected to contain them. Similar to 1. Testing with the suspected allergen(s)

1. The concentration of the allergen in the final product is too low to elicit a positive patch test reaction, but sufficient to produce a clinical dermatitis through multiple exposures or special anatomic site exposure.
2. Certain environmental factors cannot be reproduced by the test procedure (e.g. humidity, friction, temperature, etc.).

Therefore, performing special tests, such as tests with the product's extracts, repeated open application tests (ROATs), provocative use tests (PUTs), may be indicated.

The positive patch test reactions for which clinical relevance cannot be established may represent false-positive results. However, much too frequently they represent true-positive reactions wherein the patient fails to recall a significant exposure or the clinician does not retrieve the pertinent historical data, trace the responsible environmental exposure or perform the appropriate tests.

8.7
Suggestions for Improved Evidence-Based Diagnosis of Relevance

As mentioned in the preceding sections, assessing relevance is not easy. Nevertheless efforts should be undertaken to overcome those difficulties.

Table 8.6. Suggestions for improved evidence-based diagnosis of relevance

1. Re-question the patient in light of the test results
2. Perform a worksite or home visit
3. Seek cross-reacting substances
4. Consider concomitant and simultaneous sensitization
5. Consider indirect, accidental, or seasonal contact
6. Obtain information about environmental allergens from lists and textbooks
7. Obtain information from the product's manufacturer
8. Perform chemical analysis of products
9. Perform sequential tests with the allergen and the suspected products (tests with extracts, ROAT, PUT, etc.)

Suggestions for improved evidence-based diagnosis of relevance are listed in Table 8.6.

In conclusion, "The relevance of a reaction is whether it explains any dermatitis in the patient. This is a pragmatic decision strongly influenced by the knowledge, inquisitiveness and determination of the dermatologist, and the time and resources available to him or her. In difficult cases, it is an interactive process of follow-up and reassessment" [9].

References

1. Fischer TI, Hansen J, Kreilgård B, Maibach HI (1989) The science of patch test standardization. Immun Allergy Clin 9:417–434
2. Bruze M, Isaksson M, Edman B, Björkner B, Fregert S, Möller H (1995) A study on expert reading of patch test reactions: inter-individual accordance. Contact Dermatitis 32:331–337
3. de Groot AC (1999) Clinical relevance of positive patch test reactions to preservatives and fragrances. Contact Dermatitis 41:224–226
4. Lachapelle JM (1997) A proposed relevance scoring system for positive allergic patch test reactions: practical implications and limitations. Contact Dermatitis 36:39–43
5. Marks JG Jr, Belsito DV, De Leo VA, et al. (1998) North American Contact Dermatitis Group patch test results for the detection of delayed-type hypersensitivity to topical allergens. J Am Acad Dermatol 38:911–918
6. Ale SI, Maibach HI (1995) Clinical relevance in allergic contact dermatitis. Dermatosen 43:119–121
7. Ale SI, Maibach HI (2001) Operational definition of occupational allergic contact dermatitis. In: Kanerva L, Menné T, Wahlberg J, Maibach HI (eds) Handbook of occupational dermatology. Springer, Berlin Heidelberg New York, pp 344–350
8. Fregert S (1988) Physicochemical methods for detection of contact allergens. Dermatol Clin 6:97–104
9. Rycroft RJG (2002) Relevance in contact dermatitis. Contact Dermatitis 46 [Suppl 4]:39

CHAPTER 9

The True Test System

J.-M. LACHAPELLE, H. I. MAIBACH

9.1
Introduction

Conventional patch testing (as described and evaluated in other chapters of this book) is extensively used by the dermatological community throughout the world. One of the pitfalls of conventional patch testing is that allergens are not evenly dispersed in petrolatum.

True Test represents an alternative way of patch testing [1] that is intended to avoid an uneven dispersion of the allergens applied on the skin.

9.2
The True Test System

The True Test is a ready-to-use patch test system. It represents a more sophisticated approach in the technology of patch testing, taking into account the parameter of optimal penetration and delivery of allergens through the skin [2]. The allergens are incorporated in hydrophilic gels. Each gel (e.g. hydroxypropylcellulose, polyvinylpyrrolidone) is adapted to each individual allergen. The patches measure 0.81 cm² (9 mm²), and the gel is coated on a polyester sheet. For protection against light and air, the strips are contained in airtight and opaque poaches. True Test standard procedures used in manufacturing and quality control guarantee uniform quality and consistent performance [3].

The main advantage of the True Test system is that it is ready to apply and thus time-saving. Its limitations are fourfold: (a) the cost, as compared with conventional patch testing; (b) the limited number of allergens available nowadays; (c) the fact that most epidemiological studies on patch test results are based on the use of conventional patch testing; (d) the current series is very outdated.

A re-evaluation of comparative cost–benefit implications [4] of both systems could speed the move towards the widespread use of True Test in the years to come.

9.3
The Standard True Test Series

The standard True Test series consists of 24 patches (two panels), with 12 on each of two panels (Table 9.1). Each patch is coated with a thin dry film

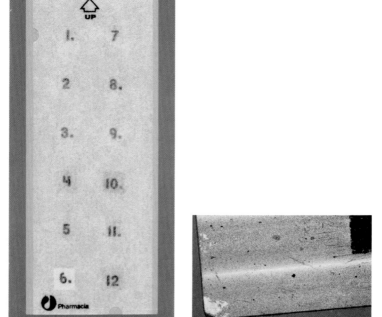

a   b

Fig. 9.1a, b. True Test. Strip: allergens 1 to 12. **b** Microscopic view of a True Test to balsam of Peru

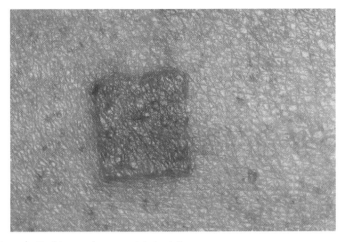

Fig. 9.1c. Positive patch test to nickel sulphate

that incorporates a specific allergen or allergen mixture in a calibrated dose (Fig. 9.1).

The amount of allergen incorporated in each test is not expressed in terms of concentrations, but in terms of micrograms/cm^2.

Investigations conducted with Panel 1 [5] and Panel 2 [6] show that results are highly reproducible.

The list of True Test standard series of allergens differs slightly from lists proposed in conventional patch testing (see Chap. 4).

A Panel 3 is under current evaluation in several centres. This panel will potentially include different allergens such as bronopol, imidazolidinylurea, diazolidinylurea, bacitracin, tixocortol-21-pivalate, budesonide, hydrocortisone-17-butyrate and others. It is designed to extend the scope of investigation of allergic patients.

Table 9.1. The standard True Test series

Allergens	($\mu g/cm^2$)
Panel 1	
1 Nickel sulphate	200
2 Wool alcohols	1,000
3 Neomycin sulphate	230
4 Potassium dichromate	23
5 Caine mix	630
6 Fragrance mix	430
7 Colophony	850
8 Epoxy resin	50
9 Quinoline mix	190
10 Balsam of Peru	800
11 Ethylenediamine dihydrochloride	50
12 Cobalt chloride	20
Panel 2	
13 *p-tert*-Butylphenol formaldehyde resin	50
14 Paraben mix	1,000
15 Carba mix	250
16 Black rubber mix	75
17 Cl+Me-Isothiazolinone (Kathon CG)	4
18 Quaternium 15	100
19 Mercaptobenzothiazole	75
20 *p*-Phenylenediamine	90
21 Formaldehyde (*N*-hydroxymethyl succinimide)	180
22 Mercapto mix	75
23 Thimerosal (thiomersal)	8
24 Thiuram mix	25

9.4
Methodology of Use

The application of True Test is as follows [7]:

a. The envelope is opened, the panel is removed, and the backing is removed from the series.

b. The adhesive backing is numbered (1–12 for series 1 and 13–24 for series 2). The series 1 panel is applied to the left back by first laying the lower edge of the adhesive backing to the back skin and then slowly applying gentle pressure with the fingers as the rest of the panel is smoothed upward.

c. The series 2 panel is applied in a similar fashion to the right upper back. The marker pen is used to mark the position of the notches on the panels.

When using True Test, the reading scores are identical to those adopted for conventional patch testing (see Sect. 3.8).

9.5
Additional Practical Information

True Test is supplied in boxes of ten standard tests (2 × 10). Advice is given to store it at +2° to +8°C. The shelf life under the above conditions is 24 months. The expiry date is stated on the package.

To assist when interpreting the results and advising the patient, True Test system includes:

a. Templates to identify each allergen
b. Patient information leaflets which answer the most commonly asked questions about the test procedure
c. A product manual to assist the physician

True Test is marketed by: Mekos Laboratories AS, Herredsvejen 2, 3400 Hillerod, Denmark (Tel.: +45-48-207100, Fax: +45-48-207101, www.mekos.dk, info@mekos.dk)

References

1. Andersen KE (2002) The interest of the True Test in patch testing. Ann Dermatol Venereol 129:1S148
2. Fischer T, Maibach HI (1985) The thin layer rapid use epicutaneous test (TRUE-Test), a new patch test method with high accuracy. Br J Dermatol 112:63–68
3. Fischer T, Kreilgard B, Maibach HI (2001) The true value of the True Test for allergic contact dermatitis. Current Allergy and Asthma Reports 1:316–322
4. Rajagopalan R, Anderson RT, Sama S (1998) An economic evaluation of patch testing in the diagnosis and management of allergic contact dermatitis. Am J Contact Dermatitis 9:149–154

5. Lachapelle JM, Bruynzeel DP, Ducombs G, Hannuksela M, Ring J, White IR, Wilkinson JD, Fischer T, Bilberg K (1988) European multicenter study of the True Test®. Contact Dermatitis 19:91–97

6. Wilkinson JD, Bruynzeel DP, Ducombs G, Frosch PJ, Gunnarsson Y, Hannuksela M, Lachapelle JM, Ring J, Shaw S, White IR (1990) European multicenter study of True Test®, Panel 2. Contact Dermatitis 22:218–225

7. Marks JG Jr, Elsner P, De Leo V (2002) Contact and occupational dermatology, 3rd edn. Mosby, St. Louis, p 47

Part 2
Prick Testing

CHAPTER 10

The Spectrum of Diseases for Which Prick Testing Is Recommended
Patients Who Should Be Investigated

J.-M. LACHAPELLE, H. I. MAIBACH

Prick tests are primarily used to detect antigens (allergens) involved in the occurrence of type I immediate skin reactions. The classic (but not exclusive) example of such reactions is immunological contact urticaria (see Fig. 10.1). This is caused by an antigen antibody, type I, immunoglobulin E (IgE)-mediated hypersensitivity reaction. The antigen is the chemical contactant that binds to specific IgE antibodies on the surface of dermal mast cells. This triggers degranulation and liberation of vasoactive substances, primarily histamine, that cause dermal oedema surrounded by an erythematous flare. Elevated serum levels of specific IgE antibodies have been demonstrated in response to contact urticariogens such as natural latex.

Prick tests will also detect non-immunological urticarial reactions provoked by substances which have a direct vasoactive (non-immunological) effect, resulting in a direct release of vasoactive molecules, which cause a localized response in almost any normal subject. These positive prick test reactions are classically observed in clinical practice, but it must be remembered that they do not represent the main purpose of prick testing.

10.1
The Contact Urticaria Syndrome

The contact urticaria syndrome (CUS), first defined as a biological entity by Maibach and Johnson [1], comprises a heterogeneous group of inflammatory reactions that usually appear within minutes after cutaneous or mucosal contact with the eliciting agent and disappear within 24 h, usually within a few hours [2, 3]. The term "syndrome" clearly illustrates the biological and clinical polymorphism of this entity, which may be either

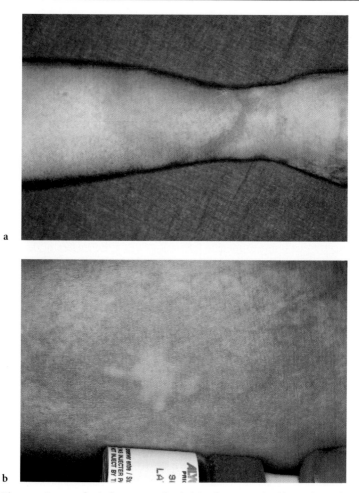

a

b

Fig. 10.1. Immunological contact urticaria (**a**) to latex proteins (from a latex glove). **b** Positive prick test reaction to latex.

localized or generalized and may involve organs other than the skin, such as the respiratory or the gastrointestinal tract, as well as the vascular system, displaying a wide spectrum of clinical manifestations, ranging from mild erythema and/or itching, to death.

Protein contact dermatitis (PCD), which could be considered a part of CUS, is described separately (see Sect. 10.2) for didactic (clinically related) reasons.

10.1.1
Clinical Symptoms and Stages of CUS

The symptoms can be classified according to morphology and severity (Table 10.1). In the mildest cases, there are only subjective symptoms (invisible contact urticaria). These are reported as itching, tingling, or burning sensations, without any objective change, or just a discrete erythema occurs. In daily practice, these reactions are seen from cosmetics and from fruits and vegetables.

Wheal and flare at the contact area is the prototype of contact urticaria (Fig. 10.1), while generalized urticaria following a local contact is less common.

Extracutaneous symptoms may also occur as part of a more severe reaction and may include rhinoconjunctivitis, asthmatic attack, and orola-

Table 10.1. The contact urticaria syndrome (CUS): staging by symptomatology (from [3])

Stage 1	Localized urticaria Dermatitis Non-specific symptoms (itching, tingling, burning etc.)
Stage 2	Generalized urticaria Cutaneous and extracutaneous reactions
Stage 3	Rhinoconjunctivitis Orolaryngeal symptoms Bronchial asthma Gastrointestinal symptoms
Stage 4	Anaphylactic symptoms

ryngeal or gastrointestinal manifestations. Finally, anaphylaxis may occur as the most severe manifestation of CUS.

Urticarial lesions of CUS do not differ clinically from those observed in common urticaria. Itching erythematous macules develop (at the site of contact) into wheals consisting of pale-pink, oedematous, raised skin areas, often with a surrounding flare. They appear in variable numbers and sizes, ranging from a few millimetres to lesions covering a large area, corresponding to the site of contact. These clinical variants are well illustrated in contact urticaria to rubber latex, a clinical entity which has exploded (in terms of numbers of cases) during the last decade.

10.1.2
Etiology and Mechanisms of CUS

The mechanisms underlying immediate-contact reactions are divided into two main types: immunological and non-immunological. However, there are substances that cause immediate contact reactions whose mechanisms (immunological or not) remain unknown [4].

Immunological Contact Urticaria

Immunological contact urticaria (ICU) is a type I hypersensitivity immunological reaction in individuals who have previously contacted the causative agent and synthesized specific immunoglobulin E (IgE) antibodies against this agent. IgE molecules react with IgE receptors on the mast cells, basophils, eosinophils, Langerhans' cells, and other cells. Eventually, allergen penetrating through the skin or mucosal membrane will react with two adjacent IgE molecules bound to the cell membranes of the mast cells. Within minutes, histamine, neutral proteases and proteoglycans are released from the mast cells, resulting in an immediate skin response. The allergen-IgE reaction also leads to synthesis of leucotrienes, prostaglandins and platelet-activating factors in the cell membranes of the activated mast cells. The mast cells also release chemotactic factors attracting eosinophils and T cells from the vessels into the dermis.

Immunological-type agents are confirmed by specific positive radioallergosorbent tests (RASTs) and by negative tests on control subjects.

The number of substances that have been reported to produce ICU is protean. Most examples refer to proteins (also responsible for protein contact dermatitis; see Fig. 10.2). Proteins can penetrate through normal human skin; any disorder in skin barrier function enhances protein penetration. Proteins are of vegetal or animal origin. The list has no limitation, since recent reports from the literature regularly provide additional urticariogens. An extensive repertoire of most common animal, plant or other derivate (natural product) proteins was recently proposed [3]. Rubber latex is by far the most common cause of ICU; several proteins have been incriminated. Due to its major importance, a special section has been devoted to latex contact urticaria (Sect. 10.1.3).

Apart from proteins, several non-protein allergens are able to provoke ICU. Among others, food-derived and food-associated materials such as preservatives, flavourings, stabilizers, emulsifiers and antioxidants also responsible for allergic contact dermatitis are often quoted [3]. Ammonium persulphate and other persulphates used in hair bleaches represent the most common cause of ICU in hairdressers (ammonium persulphate could also act as a non-immunological urticariogen).

In all these circumstances, prick testing is the investigation tool to be used in order to trace etiological factors responsible for ICU.

Non-immunological Contact Urticaria

Non-immunological contact urticaria (NICU) occurs in subjects not sensitized to the contactant, i.e. almost any normal subject. The mechanism of action is the result of a direct release of vasoactive substances, which causes a localized response. Prostaglandins are mediators in the reaction (to at least benzoic acid, sorbic acid and methylnicotinate). The NICU is often (but not always) limited to erythematous macules without oedema rather than a real wheal-and-flare reaction. In practice, the intensity of reactions depends mainly on the duration of exposure, the concentration of the contactant, and other factors such as rubbing or scratching. The reaction usually remains localized, and systemic reactions are probably not evoked. Substances capable of producing NICU are not proteins, but low-molecular-weight molecules that easily cross the skin barrier. Responsible agents include plants, animals and chemical substances. Many of the chemical substances involved are used as flavourings, fragrances, and preservatives used in the cosmetic, pharmaceutical and food industries.

As mentioned previously, prick testing reproduces experimentally NICU reactions at the site of application. Nevertheless, prick testing is not primarily aimed at tracing NICU contactants, which are well-known urticariogens. Prick testing provides positive results in almost all normal individuals.

Contact Urticaria of Uncertain Mechanism

This category is considered provisional, since it implies uncertain mechanism(s). It will be probably more precisely defined when adequate research is conducted in this field. In some instances, the reaction resembles that of ICU, but no specific IgE can be demonstrated in the patient's serum or in the tissues. It is possible that there are other immunological mechanisms in addition to the IgE-mediated ones. Specific IgG and IgM might activate the complement cascade through the classic pathway. A classic example is provided by ammonium persulphate; there have been several reports of both localized and generalized contact urticaria, as well as respiratory symptoms and even anaphylactoid reactions. Although the clinical symptoms correspond to an IgE-mediated reaction, IgE antibodies against ammonium persulphate have not been demonstrated. Similar considerations are applicable to formaldehyde.

Prick testing also detects the etiological agent(s) in cases of contact urticaria of uncertain mechanism. In such cases, the result of prick testing may also be positive in some control subjects.

10.1.3
Contact Urticaria to Natural Rubber Latex

Natural rubber latex refers to products derived from or containing the milky fluid, or natural latex, produced by the tropical rubber tree *Hevea brasiliensis*, a tree originating from the Amazon basin.

IgE-mediated natural rubber latex hypersensitivity to the constituent proteins of natural rubber latex is now recognized as a health problem of growing importance [5–7]. While the prevalence of natural rubber latex sensitization among the general population is estimated to be less than 1%, 3%–17% of healthcare workers and up to 50% of spina bifida patients are sensitized. Other high-risk groups have also been identified: patients with a history of multiple surgical interventions, atopic individuals, people working in factories where natural rubber latex is manufactured, patients suffering from hand dermatitis and patients presenting allergies to certain plant-derived food, especially "tropical" fruit. Natural rubber latex gloves (mainly but not exclusively surgical ones) represent the most common source of skin contact allergy, but many other rubber items (e.g. rubber balloons) can also be incriminated.

Natural latex is a complex mixture for which allergenicity depends on botanical, chemical, immunological and epidemiological variables. Today, several natural latex allergens have been identified and characterized at both the molecular and immunological levels. Most of those proteins are present in the lacticifer cells. In addition, several structural proteins have been described as allergens. Among these numerous proteins recognized as allergenic contactants, some are considered more important, e.g. rubber elongation factor (Hev b1), rubber elongation factor homologue (Hev b3), Hev b5, Hev b6.01, Hev b6.02, Hev b6.03, but many others may be of interest.

Diagnosis of IgE-mediated hypersensitivity to natural rubber latex is based on: (a) a clinical history of CUS (see Sect. 10.1.1), and (b) the confirmation of IgE-mediated reaction by appropriate reactions. Skin prick testing (see Chap. 11) is extensively used throughout the world and provides reasonably good sensitivity and specificity. The alternative (usually considered less performant) is the assessment of specific IgE antibodies to latex (RAST). The sensitivity of RAST was recently improved by adding Hev b5 to the solid phase. False-positive results may be due to cross-reactivity between the major allergen hevein (Hev b6.02) and class I chitinases present in various fruits such as avocado and banana [7].

Natural rubber latex hypersensitivity has become so important nowadays that, in some clinics, prick testing with natural rubber latex extract is recommended as a routine additional test to the international standard series of patch tests (see Sect. 9.5); however, some authors reserve its use only to well-defined circumstances, e.g. when clinical history is evocative or before surgery and/or other medical interventions when increased risk of contact is evident.

10.2
Protein Contact Dermatitis

Protein contact dermatitis (PCD) is a complex entity, originally described by Hjorth and Roed-Petersen [8] and accepted as a well-defined syndrome [3, 9]. Its most usual clinical presentation is hand dermatitis (described first among food handlers) that may resemble an ordinary chronic or recurrent contact dermatitis, either of the delayed allergic variety or one of chronic irritation. However, redness, wheals and sometimes microvesicles appear as symptoms of contact urticaria, usually within an hour after skin contact with the causative agent. These immediate changes usually appear only in skin sites previously affected by eczematous dermatitis.

Most often, it is not possible to depict the presence of an immediate component in hand dermatitis on the basis of the clinical examination; therefore, a detailed clinical history is essential. A distinction feature from classic allergic contact dermatitis is the fact that the patient complains of immediate symptoms such as burning, itching or stinging accompanied by redness, swelling or vesiculation when handling the allergen. To a large extent, these symptoms resemble those of skin irritation and can be misinterpreted if the patient is not questioned properly. Lesions of PCD are mainly located on hands and forearms. It has been advocated that PCD could represent a mixed situation, including both immediate (type I) and delayed (type IV) hypersensitivity reactions to allergenic proteins. Moreover, skin irritation by contactants could intervene as an additional cause. PCD is said to be common in atopic rather than in non-atopic patients, but the atopic background is not a prerequisite. In other words it may occur without any personal or family history of atopy.

Clinical variants do exist:

- Fingertip dermatitis. Mainly but not exclusively of the "gripping type" (see Sect. 2.4.2). Itching is often present, and may be distinctive.
- Chronic paronychia. This is a common variant mainly observed in patients who have chronically wet hands [10]. Wet foods are a combined source of factors, where the food may be an irritant and an allergic contactant. It is therefore predominantly a disease of domestic workers and fishmongers. Bacterial and/or *Candida albicans* infection may be associated in some cases (Fig. 10.2).

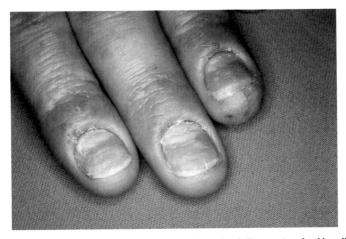

Fig. 10.2. Occupational protein contact dermatitis to food allergens in a food handler

The various clinical facets of PCD are listed in Table 10.2.

Prick testing (and its variants; see Chap. 11) is the key tool in the etiological diagnosis of PCD. The atopy patch test (see Chap. 6) could be an additional diagnostic procedure. This approach must be linked with conventional patch testing, meaningful for a complete evaluation of each individual case.

Table 10.2. Clinical facets of protein contact dermatitis (PCD)

Chronic dermatitis, mainly located on the hands and/or forearms, sharing common features with irritant and/or allergic contact dermatitis. Atopic background may be present. In that case, differential diagnosis with atopic dermatitis of the hands may be subtle and imprecise.

Urticarial symptoms (contact urticaria) are usually present, but they are often underestimated, since they are transient (acute onset after contact) and partly occulted by underlying dermatitis.

A variant of PCD is fingertip dermatitis, mainly the "gripping" form (i.e. involving thumb, index and medius of one or both hands). Itching may be a distinctive feature.

Chronic paronychia.

References

1. Maibach HI, Johnson HL (1975) Contact urticaria syndrome. Contact urticaria to diethyltoluamide (immediate-type hypersensitivity). Arch Dermatol 111: 726–730
2. von Krogh G, Maibach HI (1982) The contact urticaria syndrome. Semin Dermatol 1:59–66
3. Ale SI, Maibach HI (2000) Occupational contact urticaria. In: Kanerva L, Elsner P, Wahlberg JE, Maibach HI (eds) Handbook of occupational dermatology. Springer, Berlin Heidelberg New York, pp 200–216
4. Amin S, Lahti A, Maibach HI (1997) Contact urticaria syndrome. CRC Press, Boca Raton
5. Turjanmaa K, Palosuo T, Alenius H, et al (1997) Latex allergy diagnosis: in vivo and in vitro standardization of a natural rubber latex extract. Allergy 52:41–50
6. Ebo D (2000) IgE mediated allergy from natural rubber latex. The UCB Institute of Allergy, Brussels
7. Turjanmaa K (2002) Latex allergy. Contact Dermatitis 46 [Suppl 4]:S30
8. Hjorth N, Roed-Petersen J (1976) Occupational protein contact dermatitis in food handlers. Contact Dermatitis 2:28–42
9. Janssens V, Morren M, Dooms-Goossens A, Defreef H (1995) Protein contact dermatitis: myth or reality? Brit J Dermatol 132:1–6
10. Tosti A, Buerra L, Mozelli R (1992) Role of food in the pathogenesis of chronic paronychia. J Am Acad Dermatol 27:706–710

CHAPTER 11

The Methodology of Prick Testing and Its Variants

J.-M. LACHAPELLE, H. I. MAIBACH

As emphasized in Chap. 10, the major aim of the prick testing procedure is to trace allergenic contactants that produce immediate (type I) immunoglobulin E (IgE)-mediated hypersensitivity. Prick testing is not primarily intended to detect positive reactions to non-immunological urticariogens. On the other hand, non-immunological reactivity can make the interpretation of test results more difficult [1].

11.1
Prick Test: Technical Modalities and Reading

The prick test is usually the most convenient test method for detecting IgE-mediated allergy. Large numbers of commercial prick test allergens are available; self-made allergens can also be used (see Sect. 11.7). They are kept in a refrigerator.

11.1.1
Technique of Puncture

Drops of allergen solutions are applied to the volar aspect of the forearm or to the upper part of the back. The flexures of the elbows must be avoided, since this may give rise to not easily readable reactions, either positive or negative. Other skin sites are not convenient as well. An important point concerns the distance between the individual prick tests. These are applied ideally 3.5 cm apart, to avoid overlapping of reactions at reading. If such a distance is not respected, difficulties in correct reading are obvious and no definite conclusion can be drawn. This mistake in technology happens too often, even among well-trained clinicians.

When drops of allergen solutions are applied to the skin, they are pierced with a special lancet (e.g. the Dome-Hollister-Stier prick test lancet, the plastic lancet Stallerpoint Stallergènes, the metallic lancet Allerbiopoint Allerbio Laboratories).

Stallerpoint and Allerbiopoint are used in many European clinics. Stallerpoint (Stallergènes, 6 rue Alexis-de-Tocqueville, 92183 Antony Cedex, France) is a polymethacrylate lancet (length: 1.1 mm; four microscopic furrows allow a progressive and reproducible penetration of allergens into epidermis; presenting itself as a blister of ten sterile disposable lancets). The lancet conforms to the European Directive N93/42/CEE.

Allerbiopoint (Allerbio Laboratories, 55271 Varennes-en-Argonne Cedex, France) is a stainless steel lancet (length: 1.1 mm; penetration angle 45°; presenting itself as a blister of ten sterile disposable lancets). The lancet conforms to the European Directive N93/42/CEE.

Puncture is made by gentle pressure; some authors, when puncturing, exert a slight rotation movement to ensure better penetration of the allergen. No bleeding may occur.

11.1.2
Control Solutions

Prick testing of allergens needs the concomitant use of controls, positive and negative.

Positive Controls

- Histamine chlorhydrate solution (10 mg/ml) to measure direct reactivity to histamine
- Codeine phosphate solution (9%) to verify in each individual the aptitude for mast cell degranulation

In the dermato-allergology unit at Louvain University, Brussels, Belgium, both controls are always performed. It is our experience that positive prick tests to codeine phosphate are very uniform in all patients (with some exceptions), whereas positive prick tests to histamine chlorhydrate are more variable from patient to patient (within acceptable limits).

Negative Controls

- Saline and/or the vehicle of the allergens is used as a negative control.

11.1.3
Reading Time

After 15 min, the allergen and control droplets are wiped off with soft paper tissue. Conventional time reading is 15–20 min, since we are evaluating an immunological immediate-type I reaction.

11.1.4
Reading Prick Test Results

Reading prick test reactions (Fig. 11.1) needs careful evaluation and interpretation, taking into account several parameters of prime importance.

- The negative control ought to be negative; if positive, it raises questions about the reading of allergen prick tests. Its main interest is therefore to detect false-positive reactions.
- Wheal and flare reactions to positive controls, which appear around the piercing usually in minutes, are measured in terms of diameters and/or surface area.
- Allergen prick test results are usually expressed as the mean of the longest diameter of the wheal and the largest diameter perpendicular to it.
  Reactions greater than 3 mm and at least half of that produced by histamine are regarded as positive [2, 3]. Reactions smaller than those produced by histamine may not be clinically significant.
- If the patient has dermographism (factitious urticaria), skin piercing produces usually small (1–2 mm) wheals which may make the interpretation of the results very difficult.

There is a clear-cut difference in terms of reading between patch testing and prick testing. Patch testing is a codified procedure that does not imply any control, whereas prick testing is invariably submitted to controls either positive or negative in order to achieve correct interpretation of results.

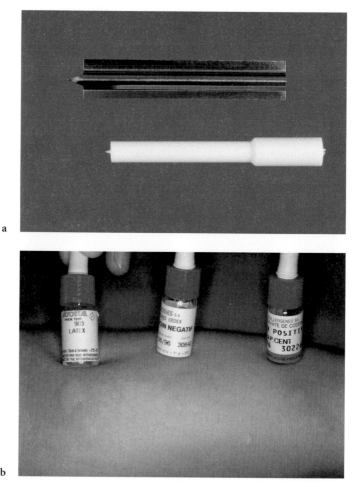

a

b

Fig. 11.1 a, b. Prick testing. **a** Prick test lancets. **b** Positive prick test to latex; positive and negative controls

The final goal in prick testing is to assess (either past or current) relevance. The practical means to conclude "likely", "possible", "doubtful" or "not traced" relevance can be copied from those described in Chap. 8.

11.1.5
Medicaments and Prick Testing

Caution must be taken when prick testing patients treated with antihistamines. Antihistamines of the so-called third generation, extensively used nowadays, abolish the immediate reactivity of the skin usually for 1–3 days. This concerns cetirizine, loratadine, fexofenadine, ebastine, mizolastine, and the newcomers desloratadine and levocetirizine. Prick testing can be performed 3 days after stopping treatment. Longer washout periods are needed with ketotifen (15 days) and astemizole (4 weeks).

Oral methylprednisolone more than 8 mg daily and equivalent doses of other corticosteroids may also weaken the immediate reactivity of the skin. Other drugs, such as anti-inflammatory non-steroid drugs as well as topical application of corticosteroids do not affect significantly prick test results.

11.1.6
False-Negative Reactions

False-negative reactions may occur. Interpretation of results needs caution:

- When reactions to positive controls are weak and/or negative
- When time reading is inadequate
- When patients are treated with antihistamines or oral corticosteroids (see Sect. 11.1.5)

11.1.7
False-Positive Reactions

False-positive reactions may occur. Interpretation of results needs caution:

- When reactions to negative controls are positive
- When patients have dermographism
- When all prick test sites react positively in a similar way

11.1.8
Prick Tests in Children and Babies

Prick tests can be performed, if suitable, in children and babies, whose skin reactivity is similar to that observed in adults.

11.2
Prick-by-Prick Test

A modification of the prick test is the prick-by-prick test, used especially for prick testing with fresh foodstuffs, e.g. fruits and vegetables [4].

A piece of food is pricked with an ordinary prick test lancet, immediately after which the skin is pricked with the same lancet. This fresh food prick testing is handy and superior to prick testing with commercial food allergens.

11.3
Scratch Test

This previously common method for detecting immediate allergy is still used when only non-standardized allergens are available. If the prick test is used for testing with non-standardized allergens, e.g. flours, edible roots, vegetables and fruits, skin infections and other untoward inflammatory processes can be produced. A scratch approximately 5 mm long is made with a blood lancet or venepuncture needle, and bleeding is avoided. The back and arms are the preferred test sites. Small amounts of allergen solution are applied to the scratches, and the results are read 15–20 min later. Powdered allergens are mixed with a drop of physiological saline or 0.1 N NaOH on the scratch. Histamine chlorohydrate 10 mg/ml is the positive, and saline or 0.1 N NaOH the negative control. Reactions equal to or greater than those from histamine are usually clinically significant.

11.4
Scratch-Chamber Test

Certain foodstuffs, e.g. edible roots, fruits and vegetables, tend to dry out too quickly when applied to a scratch. Covering the scratch with a large (inner diameter: 12 mm) Finn Chamber (Epitest, Helsinki, Finland) prevents drying out of the test material [5]. The positive and negative controls and the way results are read are the same as for the scratch test.

11.5
Comparative Indications of Prick Testing and Other Related Tests

The indications for which the use of prick tests and other related tests are advised are listed in Table 11.1.

Table 11.1. Comparative indications of prick tests and other related tests (from [1])

Test	Indications
Prick test	For IgE-mediated allergy; especially for standardized allergen solutions
Prick-by-prick	Recommended for testing with fresh foods
Scratch test	For IgE-mediated immediate allergy; non-standardized allergen can also be used
Scratch-chamber test	Especially for testing foodstuffs

11.6
Intradermal Testing

Nowadays, as far as the etiological diagnosis of CUS and/or PCD is concerned, prick testing and its variants do not have to be complemented by intradermal testing. Intradermal testing with rubber latex extracts has been practised in some studies, but it is no longer advised. Therefore, in practice, the use of intradermal testing is limited to investigations in relation with drug eruptions (see Chap. 12).

11.7
Prick Testing: Allergens of Interest for Skin Problems

Many categories of standardized allergens are available for prick testing; there is no standard series (compared with patch testing). Among the long list quoted in catalogues, some are of greater importance as far as skin problems are concerned. A few series are listed below.

11.7.1
Latex

Natural rubber latex glove extracts have been widely used as skin prick test allergens. However, since the allergen content of natural rubber latex gloves varies considerably, it is of extreme importance to dispose of the most suitable glove for test material. An updated list on the allergenicity of natural rubber latex gloves is available from the National Agency for Medicines, Medical Device Centre (P.O. Box 278, 00531 Helsinki, Finland). For the time being, only one standardized commercial natural rubber latex extract is available in Europe (Stallergènes, 6 rue Alexis-de-Tocqueville, 92183 Antony Cedex, France) [6]. In addition, a few non-standardized skin prick test extracts (ALK-Abello a/s, Hörsholm, Denmark; Bencard, Missisanga, Ontario, Canada) are commercialized in Europe and Canada. Turjanmaa et al. [7] studied Stallergènes, ALK, Bencard, and a home-made extract, and observed a sensitivity of 83%, 54%, 92% and 92% respectively.

No U.S. Food and Drug Administration-approved commercial skin test extract allergen is currently available in the USA.

Cross-sensitization may occur with plant-derived food allergens, especially "tropical" fruits. Well-known cross-reactive foods include avocado, banana, chestnut, kiwi, papaya, potato and peaches ("latex-fruit syndrome"). There is also serologic cross-reactivity between natural rubber latex and aeroallergens, e.g. pollen ("latex-mould syndrome").

11.7.2
Airborne Environmental per Annum Allergens

The most common airborne environmental per annum allergens (the list is not limited) are quoted in Table 11.2.

In terms of quality, this group is very heterogeneous. Allergens from mites and cockroaches have a good specificity and sensitivity. Sensitivity is less accurate for mould (except *Alternaria*)) and animal allergens.

In atopic patients, prick testing with mite allergens competes with the atopy patch test (see Chap. 6); further studies may reveal their complementarity.

11.7.3
Airborne Environmental Seasonal Allergens

The most common airborne environmental seasonal allergens (the list is not limited) are quoted in Table 11.3. These allergens are pollens from dif-

Table 11.2. Airborne environmental per annum allergens

Mites	From house dust: *Dermatophagoides farinae, Dermatophagoides pteronyssinus, Euroglyphus maynei* From storage: *Acarus siro, Glycyphagus domesticus, Lepidoglyphus destructor, Tyrophagus putrescenciae*
Animals	Cat, dog, horse, guinea pig, hamster, rabbit, feathers
Domestic insects	Cockroaches
Moulds	*Alternaria, Aspergillus, Botrytis, Chaetomium, Cladosporium, Epicoccum, Merulius, Mucor, Penicillium, Pullularia, Rhizopus, Stemphyllium, Trichotecium*

Table 11.3. Airborne environmental seasonal allergens (pollens)

Trees	Betulaceae: birch, hazel, elm, alder Fagaceae: chestnut, oak, beech Olacaceae: olive tree, ash, privet, forsythia, lilac Cupressaceae: cypress, juniper Salicaceae: poplar, willow
Graminaceae	Fodder crops: agrostis, creeping wheat-grass, dactylis, fescue, holcus, darnel, meadow (spear)grass, phleum Cereal crops: oat, corn, maize, barley, rye
Herbaceae	Compositae: artemisia, ambrosia Chinopodiaceae: cherropodium Urticaceae: pellitory

ferent plants and are of limited interest in dermato-allergology; nevertheless, they could prove useful in atopics. They are of no use in small children, since sensitization to pollens does occur significantly at the age of
5 years. They are chosen according to the geographical area, in relation
with environmental variations.

11.7.4
Food Allergens (Trophallergens)

The interest of prick testing with foodstuffs is primordial when protein
contact dermatitis (see Sect. 10.2) is suspected in food handlers. It is
of prime importance in occupational dermatology, when patients are
handling food repeatedly at work, e.g. bakers, bartenders, butchers, cooks,
fishermen and fishmongers.

In some cases, positive reactions can lead to a change of job; nevertheless, it is advisable to take into consideration different points of dis-
cussion (see below) before drawing any definite conclusion.

The quality of food allergens in terms of sensitivity and specificity is
variable. It is often advisable to prick test with fresh foodstuffs, e.g. fruits
and vegetables, which are handy and more reliable, compared to commercial food allergens. Prick-by-prick testing (see Sect. 11.2), scratch testing
(Sect. 11.3) and scratch-chamber testing (Sect. 11.4) are highly recommended.

Table 11.4. Cross-sensitization potential reactions to food allergens (trophallergens)

Cereals: corn, rye, barley, oat, maize, pollens of Graminaceae
Leguminosae: peanut, soya bean, peas, lentil, broad bean, kidney bean (bush bean)
Umbelliferae: celery, carrot, parsley, fennel, anise, coriander, cumin, green pepper
Cruciferae: mustard, cabbage, cress, broccoli, turnip, radish, horseradish
Solanaceae: tomato, sweet pepper, potato, paprika, coffee, aubergine
Liliaceae (*amaryllidaceae*): garlic, onion, asparagus, chives, shallot
Nuts: walnut, coconut, hazelnut, pistachio nut, almond, cashew nut
Rutaceae: orange, lemon, grapefruit, mandarin
Drupaceae: apple, hazel nut, peach, pear, apricot, plum, raspberry, strawberry, almond, cherry, birch and hazel tree pollens
Eggs, chicken, turkey, quail, goose, pigeon, feathers
Milk, cheese, beef
Fishes
Shellfish
Mollusca
Celery, carrot, spices, artemisia
Melon, banana
Celery, birch, water melon, cucumber, ambrosia
Honey, pollens
Pork, cat (epithelia)
Latex (see Sect. 11.7.1)
Snail, mites
Barm

A pitfall when reading prick tests to foodstuffs is related to the fact that some of them may release histamine (or other vasoactive molecules).

When interpreting prick test results, cross-sensitization between foodstuffs is taken into account, but the relevance of cross-sensitization is sometimes doubtful; caution and moderation are needed when expressing our opinion to patients.

A positive prick test (or its variants) needs to be confirmed for assessment of relevance by additional procedures (anamnestic data, oral provocation test, eviction/reintroduction, etc.). This step is important prior to edict eviction measures.

Cross-sensitization reactions between food allergens (trophallergens) are listed in Table 11.4.

11.7.5
Occupational Allergens

Occupational allergens are extremely varied [8]. It is out of the scope of this book to include a list of all allergens quoted in recent years. Important ones are given in Table 11.5. Most of these allergens are not marketed as such. Therefore, they are prepared extemporaneously at the proper concentration (see textbooks) at the patch and prick test clinic.

11.7.6
Fungi

- *Malassezia furfur*
- *Candida albicans*
- *Epidermophyton*
- *Trichophyton*

Prick testing with these allergens is of very limited clinical interest. Its use is not routinely recommended.

11.7.7
Miscellaneous (Immunological and/or Non-immunological) Urticariogens

A multitude of other (immunological and/or non-immunological) urticariogens are encountered in our environment. As examples we name: blood, caterpillars, corals, jellyfish, saliva and seminal fluid.

Table 11.5. Occupational allergens

Latex (see Sect. 11.7.1)

Per annum and seasonal (pollens) allergens (see Sects. 11.7.2 and 11.7.3)

Foodstuffs (Sect. 11.7.4)

Enzymes: α amylase (bakers), cellulase, papain, xylanase

Brucella abortus, placenta (cow), amniotic fluid (veterinarians)

Silk

Pearl oysters

Urine (mice, rat)

Worms

Various plants (e.g. camomile, tulips)

Plants derivates: abietic acid, colophony, cornstarch

Tropical woods

Teak

Tobacco

Topical drugs (mainly antibiotics)

Ammonium persulphate and other persulphates

Paraphenylenediamine, para-aminophenol, paramethylaminophenol

Cosmetics, preservatives

Acrylic monomers

Carbamates

Carbonless copy paper

Diglycidyl ether of bisphenol

Formaldehyde resin

Metals (e.g. chromium salts, cobalt, nickel, platinum salts)

Epoxy resins, reactive diluents and hardeners

References

1. Hannuksela M (2001) Skin tests for immediate hypersensitivity. In: Rycroft RJG, Menné T, Frosch PJ, Lepoittevin JP (eds) Textbook of contact dermatitis, 3rd edn. Springer, Berlin Heidelberg New York, pp 519–525
2. Basomba A, Sastre A, Pelaez A, Romar A, Campos A, Garcia-Villamanzo A (1985) Standardization of the prick test. A comparative study of three methods. Allergy 40:395–399
3. Malling HJ (1985) Reproducibility of skin sensitivity using a quantitative skin prick test. Allergy 40:400–404
4. Dreborg S, Foucard T (1983) Allergy to apple, carrot and potato in children with birch pollen allergy. Allergy 38:167–172
6. Hannuksela M, Lahti A (1977) Immediate reactions to fruits and vegetables. Contact Dermatitis 3:79–84
7. Turjanmaa K, Palosuo T, Alenius H, et al (1997) Latex allergy diagnosis: in vivo and in vitro standardization of a natural rubber latex extract. Allergy 52:41–50
8. Turjanmaa K, Alenius H, Mäkinen-Kiljunen S, et al (1995) Commercial skin prick test preparations in the diagnosis of rubber latex allergy (abstract) J Allergy Clin Immunol 93:S299
9. Ale SI, Maibach HI (2000) Occupational contact urticaria. In: Kanerva L, Elsner P, Wahlberg JE, Maibach HI (eds) Handbook of occupational dermatology. Springer, Berlin Heidelberg New York, pp 200–216

Part 3
Testing in Cutaneous Systemic
Drug Reactions:
Interest and Limitations

Chapter 12

Testing Procedures in Cutaneous Adverse Drug Reactions

J.-M. Lachapelle, H. I. Maibach

12.1
General Considerations

Cutaneous adverse drug reactions (CADRs) to systemically administered drugs have increased in number during the last few years. This is due to the expanding number of new active molecules used in the treatment of a variety of diseases. CADR are varied and described in full detail in oriented manuals of dermatology [1–3].

Diagnosis of CADR may be straightforward in some cases, but less obvious in others. The link between the occurrence of a CADR and the systemic administration of a drug (considered to be the culprit agent) is sometimes difficult to assess. The problem is even more complex when several drugs are administrated concomitantly. Several criteria can be taken into account to find the relationship between drug administration and the occurrence of CADRs.

A careful analysis of such criteria has led French authors [4, 5] to describe a scale of imputation (or imputability). This scale includes intrinsic and extrinsic factors. Intrinsic factors are chronological and semeiological, whereas extrinsic ones are based on literature survey. The procedure of evaluation is rather complicated and needs experience. Its detailed description does not fit within the scope of this book. When correctly applied, it provides useful information; its use is highly recommended when CADRs to new drugs are reported. Thus far, its routine adoption has not been reached worldwide.

Table 12.1. CADR: tools of investigation for assessment of drug imputation

Clinical examination	Clinical symptoms are characteristic (or not) of a well-defined variety of CADR.
Chronological criteria	Anamnestic data are of crucial importance. Theoretically, there is a chronological link between the administration of a drug and the occurrence of CADR, and, in the same way, between the withdrawal of the drug and the resolution of CADR. Such a time schedule suffers some exceptions. Fading of clinical symptoms may occur several weeks after withdrawal of the drug.
Evaluation of additional events	Some occasional events may favour the clinical expression of CADR. These include viral infections (cytomegalovirus, Epstein-Barr virus, parvovirus B19, hepatitis B and C viruses; serological tests may be advised), immunological status, drug interference.
Skin biopsy: histopathological signs	Skin biopsy may be a contributory tool in some cases of CADR. Histopathological signs of CADR include: vacuolar alteration and clefts along the dermo-epidermal junction; accumulation of epidermal and/or dermal colloid (Civatte's) bodies; melanin pigmentary incontinence; interface lymphocytic infiltrate; presence of eosinophils. Typical pictures mainly refer to fixed (bullous and non-bullous) drug eruptions, lichenoid and psoriasiform drug eruptions, acute generalized exanthematic pustulosis. In eczematous CADR, histopathological signs are similar to those encountered in other types of eczema. Some CADRs (e.g. erythema multiforme, Stevens-Johnson syndrome, Lyell's syndrome, leucocytoclastic vasculitis) display characteristic histopathological features.
Careful check of the literature	Checking the current literature referring to CADR is a tool of prime importance. This approach includes modern routes of investigation, such as Medline, the Internet. etc.

12.2
Tools of Investigation in CADR

The link between the occurrence of a CADR and the implication of one (or more) suspected drug(s) is a difficult task for the clinician. It implies the use of several tools of investigation, listed in Table 12.1. It is important to put together the various sources of information, in order to reach a high level of imputability, the spirit of which is similar to the determination of a relevance score in patch testing (and other testing) procedures, as explained in Chap. 8.

Table 12.1 (continued)

| Testing procedures | When evaluating the imputation of a drug in the occurrence of CADR, testing (patch and/or prick) procedures can play an undisputed role (see Sects. 12.3 and 12.4), but they are only one of the pieces of the jigsaw puzzle among the other available tools of investigation. Their limitations are linked to several factors, as detailed below. |
| Provocation test | When a CADR has faded, the systemic reintroduction of the suspected drug (at a lower dose) provokes a recurrent eruption when a positive relationship does exist between the rash and the drug. This procedure provides the more accurate etiological diagnosis; it is the best tool at our disposal nowadays, but it may be submitted to ethical approval in some countries. |

CADR, cutaneous adverse drug reactions.

12.3
Patch Testing In CADR

The use of patch testing in CADR has led to many publications. A general review of the subject has been made by Bruynzeel [6]. Generally speaking, insufficient standardization in patch testing procedures is evident. Most publications refer to individual cases; extended series of positive and/or negative patch test results referring to various drugs are lacking. It is noteworthy that more publications are devoted to positive results rather than to negative ones; this is the reason why a Working Party of the European Society for Contact Dermatitis (ESCD) for the study of skin testing in investigating CADR was created. The members of the Working Party have defined some guidelines for performing skin patch tests in CADR [7].

12.3.1
The Spectrum of CADRs for Which Patch Testing Is Recommended

Positive patch test reactions can be expected to occur when the pathomechanisms of CADR involve delayed-type hypersensitivity (type IV according to the classification of Gell and Coombs) (Fig. 12.1).

As emphasized earlier (Sect. 2.3.3.2), patch tests are usually positive when systemic reactivation of allergic contact dermatitis (SRCD) occurs, i.e. baboon syndrome or Fisher's systemic contact dermatitis.

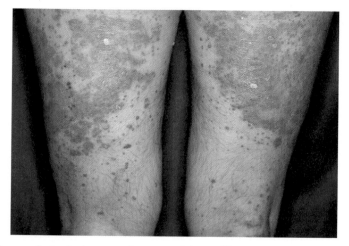

Fig. 12.1. Systemic drug eruption to a sulphonamide: eczematous symmetrical rash on the thighs

Table 12.2. A list of CADRs for which patch testing is recommended

Acute generalized exanthematic pustulosis (AGEP)
Eczematous eruptions (with no previous contact of the allergen with the skin)
Exanthematous eruptions (Fig. 12.1)
Exfoliative dermatitis or erythroderma
Fixed drug eruption (bullous or non-bullous) (Fig. 12.2)
Granulomatous drug eruption [3]
Hypersensitivity syndrome (DRESS)
Lichenoid drug eruptions
Photosensitivity (photoallergic drug eruptions); note that in this case photopatch testing is required (see Chap. 5)
Pityriasis rosea-like eruptions
Pseudolymphomatous drug eruptions
Psoriasiform drug eruptions
Systemic reactivation of allergic contact dermatitis (baboon syndrome, Fisher's systemic contact dermatitis)

Some CADR probably express a type IV reaction exclusively (e.g. maculopapular rash or eczematous reactions), whereas some others involve type I plus type IV reactions, or more complex immunological mechanisms (e.g. erythema multiforme, Stevens-Johnson syndrome).

A list of CADRs for which patch testing is recommended is presented in Table 12.2.

12.3.2
The Spectrum of CADRs for Which Patch Testing Can Be Performed (Being Still Controversial)

Some CADRs implying complex immunological pathomechanisms have been shown to provide positive patch test reactions [6, 7]. A list of CADRs for which patch testing can be performed is presented in Table 12.3.

Table 12.3. A list of CADRs for which patch testing can be performed (still controversial)

Erythema multiforme
Purpura
Stevens-Johnson syndrome
Toxic epidermal necrolysis (Lyell's syndrome)
Vasculitis

12.3.3
The Spectrum of CADRs for Which Patch Testing Is of No Interest

In some CADRs, patch testing has no practical interest. These include acne-like eruptions, alopecia (and hypotrichosis), exacerbation of psoriasis, hypertrichosis, lupus erythematosus, nail changes due to drugs, pigmentary disorders, scleroderma-like reactions, urticarial reactions and vesiculo-bullous eruptions (drug-induced pemphigoid, drug-induced pemphigus and linear IgA drug-induced bullous dermatosis).

12.3.4
Guidelines in Drug Patch Testing: General Rules

Some general principles should be borne in mind when patch testing in CADR [7]:

- An informed patient consent is needed.
- Patch tests should be performed 6 weeks to 6 months after complete healing of CDAR and at least 1 month after discontinuation of systemic corticosteroids or other immunosuppressive drugs.
- Patch tests should be performed with the commercialized drug and, whenever possible, also with the pure active products and excipients (vehicles).
- Patch testing with drugs, sharing a similar chemical structure, or from the same pharmacological family, may also be important to detect cross-sensitization (see Sect. 3.13) [8].

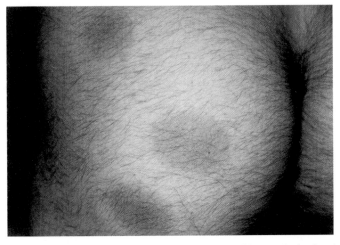

Fig. 12.2. Fixed drug eruption to piroxicam: three typical lesions (72 h after drug intake) on a buttock

- An immediate reading of patch tests (at 20 min) is advised to check the potential occurrence of an urticarial reaction. Readings are made at day 2, day 4 and day 7.
- In fixed drug eruptions (Fig. 12.2), patch tests should be performed both on normal skin and on the residual pigmented site of the fixed drug eruption. It is classically observed that patch testing gives a positive response at the site of the lesion ("local memory") and not on intact skin (Fig. 12.3).

12.3.5
Technical Aspects of Drug Patch Testing

All information referring to patch test technology, as provided in Chap. 3, is applicable to patch testing in CADR. Nevertheless, additional information regarding particular aspects of the technology is required.

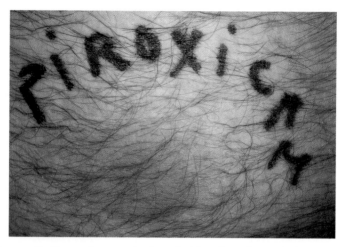

Fig. 12.3. Positive patch test to piroxicam (72 h) performed 2 months later at a previous site of fixed drug eruption

Patch Testing with Marketed Drugs: Concentrations and Vehicles

The marketed drug used by the patient can be tested (in particular when the pure drug is not available). Pills should have their coating removed, then be ground to a very fine powder. As advised by Barbaud et al. [9], this powder is incorporated at 30% in white petrolatum and diluted at 30% in water.

The powder contained in capsules is dispersed at 30% in petrolatum and/or diluted at 30% in water. The gel jacket portion of the capsules should be moistened and tested as is.

Liquid preparations are tested both as is and diluted at 30% in water. These concentrations are arbitrary, but are considered practical and useful by the members of the ESCD Working Party.

Patch Testing with Pure Substances: Concentrations and Vehicles

Whenever possible, the pure drug obtained from the manufacturer should be tested dispersed at 10% in petrolatum and also diluted at 10% in water and/or ethanol. This procedure can be adapted; concentrations and vehicles previously considered most adequate for certain drugs should also be chosen.

A complete investigation should include patch testing with preservatives, colouring agents and excipients, as is or dispersed at 10% in petrolatum or in the vehicles usually recommended for testing in allergic contact dermatitis.

Some improvements are still needed in this field of patch testing, in terms of concentrations and vehicles, in order to enhance the penetration into the skin of each individual drug. At present, we are at a craftsman's stage; improvements require scientific involvement based on multicentric studies and new technologies.

12.3.6
False-Negative Patch Test Reactions

False-negative reactions can be related to two main reasons:

- The insufficient penetration of the drug into the skin in order to elicit an allergic response.
- The allergen is not the drug itself, but one of its metabolites. The metabolites are delivered into the skin, when the drug is administered systemically, but not necessarily when the drug is applied onto the skin (depending on the enzymatic pathways involved).

12.3.7
False-Positive Patch-Test Reactions

Application of the drug onto the skin can induce a false-positive reaction (due to an irritant effect). When a new drug is patch tested (therefore, without drug reference from the literature) and gives a positive response, the interpretation of which being difficult, it is useful to patch test control subjects. Patch testing control subjects may require ethical approval.

12.4
Prick Testing in CADR

Prick testing is not currently practised in CADR. Its interest is limited to the rare cases of immunological drug urticaria.

It is advised to use pure drugs at sequential dilutions (10^{-3}, 10^{-2}, 10^{-1}, then pure) [7]. Technological aspects are similar to those described in Chap. 11.

References

1. Breathnach SM, Hinter H (1992) Adverse drug reactions and the skin. Blackwell Scientific Publications, Oxford
2. Zürcher K, Krebs A (1992) Cutaneous drug reactions. An integral synopsis of today's systemic drugs, 2nd edn. Karger, Basel
3. Bruinsma W (2000) A guide to drug eruptions. Side effects in dermatology, 7th edn. IMP, Amsterdam, Rotterdam
4. Bégaud B, Evreux JC, Jouglard J, Lagier G (1985) Unexpected or toxic drug reaction assessment (imputation). Actualization of the method used in France. Thérapie 40:111–118
5. Moore N, Paux G, Begaud B, Biour M, Loupi E, Boismare F, Royer RJ (1985) Adverse drug reaction monitoring: doing it the French way. Lancet ii:1056–1058
6. Bruynzeel D (2001) Patch testing in adverse drug reactions. In: Rycroft RJG, Menné T, Frosch P, Lepoittevin JP (eds) Textbook of contact dermatitis, 3rd edn. Springer, Berlin Heidelberg New York, pp 479–493
7. Barbaud A, Gonçalo M, Bruynzeel D, Bircher A (2001) Guidelines for performing skin tests with drugs in the investigation of cutaneous adverse drug reactions. Contact Dermatitis 45:321–328
8. Oliveira HS, Gonçalo M, Reis JP, Figueiredo A (1999) Fixed drug eruption to piroxicam. Positive patch tests with cross-sensitivity to tenoxicam. J Dermatol Treatment 10:209–212
9. Barbaud A, Reichert-Penetrat S, Trechot P, Jacquin-Petit MA, Ehlinger A, Noirez V, Faure GC, Schmutz JL, Bene MC (1998) The use of skin testing in the investigation of cutaneous adverse reactions. Br J Dermatol 139:49–58

Suggested Reading

J.-M. Lachapelle, H. I. Maibach

1. Adams RM (1990) Occupational skin disease, 2nd edn. WB Saunders Company, Philadelphia, PA, USA
2. Angelini G, Vena GA (1997) Dermatologia professionale e ambientale. ISED, Brescia, Italy
3. Breathnach SM, Hintner H (1992) Adverse drug reactions and the skin. Blackwell Scientific Publications, Oxford
4. Bruinsma W (2000) A guide to drug eruptions. Side effects in dermatology, 7th edn. IMP, Amsterdam, Rotterdam
5. Champion RH, Burton JL, Burns DA, Breathnach SM (1998) Rook/Wilkinson/Ebling Textbook of Dermatology. Blackwell Science, Oxford
6. Cronin E (1980) Contact dermatitis. Churchill Livingstone, Edinburgh
7. de Groot AC (1994) Patch testing. Test concentrations and vehicles for 3700 chemicals. Elsevier, Amsterdam
8. Elsner P, Lachapelle JM, Wahlberg JE, Maibach HI (1995) Prevention of contact dermatitis. Current problems in dermatology, vol 25. Karger, Basel
9. Foussereau J, Benezra C, Maibach HI (1982) Occupational contact dermatitis: clinical and chemical aspects. Munksgaard, Copenhagen
10. Fregert S (1981) Manual of contact dermatitis, 2nd edn. Munksgaard, Copenhagen
11. Frosch PJ, Dooms-Goossens A, Lachapelle JM, Rycroft RJG, Scheper R (1989) Current topics in contact dermatitis. Springer, Berlin Heidelberg New York
12. Hogan DJ (1994) Occupational skin disorders. Ikagu-Shoin, New York
13. Kanerva L, Elsner P, Wahlberg JE, Maibach HI (2000) Handbook of occupational dermatology. Springer, Berlin Heidelberg New York
14. Lachapelle JM, Frimat P, Tennstedt D, Ducombs G (1992) Précis de dermatologie professionnelle et de l'environnement. Masson, Paris
15. Lachapelle JM, Tennstedt D (2001) Progrès en dermato-allergologie, Bruxelles, 2001. John Libbey Eurotext, Montrouge
16. Lepoittevin JP, Basketter DA, Goossens A, Karlberg AT (1998) Allergic contact dermatitis. The molecular basis. Springer, Berlin Heidelberg New York
17. Lovell CR (1993) Plants and the skin. Blackwell Scientific Publications, Oxford

18. Malten KE, Nater JP, van Ketel WG (1976) Patch testing guidelines. Dekker and van de Vegt, Nijmegen

19. Marks JG, Elsner P, de Leo V (2002) Contact and occupational dermatology, 3rd edn. Mosby, St. Louis, MO

20. Mellström GA, Wahlberg JE, Maibach HI (1994) Protective gloves for occupational use. CRC Press, Boca Raton, FL

21. Menné T, Maibach HI (1991) Exogenous dermatoses: environmental dermatitis. CRC Press, Boca Raton, FL

22. Menné T, Maibach HI (2000) Hand eczema, 2nd edn. CRC Press, Boca Raton, FL

23. Rietschel RL, Fowler JF Jr (2000) Fisher's contact dermatitis, 5th edn. Lippincott, Williams & Wilkins, Philadelphia, PA

24. Rycroft RJG, Menné T, Frosch PJ, Lepoittevin JP (2001) Textbook of contact dermatitis, 3rd edn. Springer, Berlin Heidelberg New York

25. van der Valk PGM, Maibach HI (1995) The irritant contact dermatitis syndrome. CRC Press, Boca Raton, FL

26. Zürcher K, Krebs A (1992) Cutaneous drug reactions. An integral synopsis of today's systemic drugs. Karger, Basel

Subject Index